ENTREPRENEURING

A NURSE'S GUIDE TO STARTING A BUSINESS

GERRY VOGEL
NANCY DOLEYSH

Pub. No. 41-2201

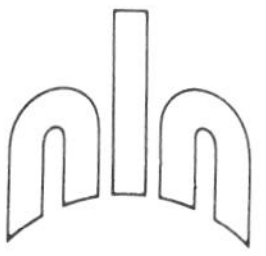

National League for Nursing • New York

The views expressed in this book reflect those of the authors and do not necessarily reflect the official views of the National League for Nursing.

ISBN 0-88737-385-2

Manufactured in the United States of America.

PREFACE

Entrepreneuring is the new frontier in nursing. If you are a nurse entrepreneur, a nurse who is intrigued by the possibility of becoming one, or a student who is interested in learning more about this emerging trend, you will find information, encouragement, and direction in this book. We are two nurses, each of whom have established successful businesses, and we want to share what we have learned with you. The key elements of this book are:

- a clear, step-by-step guide for developing and maintaining your own business,
- self-discovery and assessment exercises to help you make entrepreneurial and business decisions,
- case studies of successful nurse entrepreneurs to illustrate major points,
- an examination of the theory, process, and business aspects of a nurse consulting practice,
- application of a quality-assurance process to entrepreneurial endeavors,
- a unique nursing orientation to entrepreneuring and consulting information,
- an exploration of the many contributions nurse entrepreneurs are making to patients, other nurses, and the profession.

The information in this book represents the knowledge we gained as new entrepreneurs through a trial and error method. During our business start-up periods, we both experienced frustration because information sources were difficult to locate, widely dispersed, and lacking in information essential for nurse entrepreneurs. In the early days, working without a peer group left us feeling isolated. When we met and began to share experiences and information, we discovered new insights and developed a sense of professional support.

Our idea for this book grew out of the realization that other nurses could benefit from what we had learned, perhaps avoid some of the pitfalls, and reaffirm their professional identity through contact with a network of nurse entrepreneurs. We integrated our experiences, the experiences of the over 60 nurse entrepreneurs who contributed to the case studies, and information gathered from a variety of sources on entrepreneuring, consulting, business development, and marketing to provide a reference that is both informative and practical.

ABOUT THE AUTHORS

Since this book is our professional contact with you, we would like to tell you about ourselves and our businesses. Some things we have in common are the factors that motivated us to become entrepreneurs. Both of us had a desire for independence, flexibility, and the idea of a work focus that promoted those goals piqued our interest. In addition, we felt we could have a greater impact on the quality of nursing if we worked in an independent role.

Our businesses reflect both our experiences and professional interests. Advanced Health Care Concepts, whose president is Nancy Doleysh, MSN, RN, began as a partnership in 1980 and became a sole proprietorship in 1981. Its goal is to provide advanced clinical expertise to clients, both individuals and organizations, so they can resolve problems created by the escalating complexity and specialization in health care. For example, when a hospital decided to expand and market its orthopaedic specialty service, Doleysh helped develop policies and procedures, educate staff, coordinate support systems, including equipment, transport, and diagnostic services, and acted as preceptor to the nursing staff. Another part of her role included marketing this improved service to physicians. Her work made the organization's goal operational in a cost-effective way and had a direct positive impact on patient care.

Doleysh provides "expertise on demand" to clients, and the excitement lies in the challenge of finding new approaches and solutions to both old and evolving health care problems. She is able to use her past experiences as an educator, manager, and clinical specialist in ways that are challenging for her.

WORKSTYLES, whose director is Gerry Vogel, MSN, RN, has a different business emphasis because of the special interests of its owner. WORKSTYLES was established in 1983 as a sole proprietorship. While it provides consulting services for a variety of management problems, process-management problems are its specialty because they are the most challenging and rewarding to resolve. As a process management consultant, Vogel helps both managers and staff develop the interpersonal competencies essential for quality, productivity, and effective change.

Vogel believes that each individual brings a unique personal style to his or her work roles. These styles can be enhanced so that individuals and groups can improve their interpersonal skills and increase their effectiveness as a team. The improved group dynamics result in a collaborative, efficient team and this, in turn, improves both patient care and staff morale. Vogel's past experiences as staff nurse, educator, and administrator enable her to help clients find solutions to the problems generated in their highly competitive, fast-paced, and conflict-prone environments.

WORKSTYLES has grown since its 1983 start. In addition to organizational consulting, it presents workshops and seminars on a variety of management topics, plus providing career planning counseling to individuals.

WHAT THIS BOOK WILL DO FOR YOU

Now that we have described our businesses, we want to tell you how this book can enhance your efforts at entrepreneuring. If you have thought of starting your own business but hesitated because the barriers seemed insurmountable, this book will help you remove those barriers or, at least, reduce them to a manageable size.

The format of this book mirrors the development stages you will experience as a nurse entrepreneur. In Part I, the exploration stage, we identify the essential components of a successful entrepreneurial career move. Self-discovery tools help you with personal assessment. We present initial pre-planning strategies, and suggest ways you can maximize success.

We address the business development activities—planning, organizing, financing, marketing, and growing—in Part II. We utilize planning and decision-making tools to help you develop a systematic process for nurturing new or existing business ventures.

We present a framework for consulting in Part III. We explain general principles of consulting and the application of those principles within an organization.

In Part IV, we discuss the unique contributions that nurse entrepreneurs are making. This celebration of nursing is based on the information that our case study contributors shared with us. The stories of these nurse entrepreneurs highlight the variety, challenges, and possibilities in entrepreneurship that await you.

We wrote this book to help you take advantage of those possibilities. We dedicate this work to our nursing colleagues interested in entrepreneuring with the hope that it serves as a source of support, encouragement, and information.

Nancy Doleysh, MSN, RN,
President
Advanced Health Care Concepts

Gerry Vogel, MSN, RN
Director
WORKSTYLES

CONTENTS

Part I Entrepreneurship 1

Chapter 1 Entrepreneurial Roles 3

Definitions 3
Trends affecting entrepreneurial roles 4
Advantages and disadvantages 16

Chapter 2 Characteristics of Successful Entrepreneurs 23

Entrepreneurs' career path.. 23
The entrepreneurial personality 26
Gender differences.. 32
Entrepreneurial self-assessment.. 35

Chapter 3 Finding a Niche 55

Developing a business idea 56
Market-service analysis 70
Market testing... 85
Launching a trial balloon... 98
Self-help tips 100

Part II Establishing a Business: Ready, Set, Grow 103

Chapter 4 Planning a New Business.................................. 105

The business plan.. 105
Planning issues affecting nurse entrepreneurs 113
Research and resources.. 115

Chapter 5 Organizing a Business Start-Up 123

Organizing decisions 123
Developing a business philosophy 123

Goals as an organizing strategy ... 127
Choosing a business form ... 127
Creating a business image ... 133
Selēcting a business name ... 135
Locating a space for the business ... 138
Support and equipment services ... 141
Selecting office supplies and equipment ... 143
Establishing a work process ... 146
Developing an organized documentation process ... 148
A final look at organizing ... 150

Chapter 6 Marketing a Nursing Business ... 153

Basic marketing concepts ... 153
Promotion strategies ... 160
The marketing plan ... 168

Chapter 7 Financing a Business ... 173

Sources of start-up financing ... 173
Managing business finances ... 182
Common financial mistakes ... 207

Chapter 8 Survival and Growth ... 209

Planning the pace of growth ... 209
Managing quality assurance ... 210
Directions for small business growth ... 214
Managing growth finances ... 216

Part III The Nurse Entrepreneur As Consultant ... 221

Chapter 9 Consulting ... 223

Stages of a consulting assignment ... 223
Nurse consultant roles ... 228
Skills of the successful consultant ... 231
Documents that organize a consulting practice ... 233

Chapter 10 The Nurse As Organizational Consultant ... 241

Organizational analysis ... 241
Organizational change process ... 248
Assessment of organizational culture ... 254

Part IV The Unique Contributions of Nurse Entrepreneurs 257

Chapter 11 Enhancing Nursing through Entrepreneurship 259

Contributions to patients.. 259
Contributions to nurses and nursing 261

References.. 265

Appendix

A Nurse Entrepreneurs Who Contributed to This Book........... A1
B Business Plan: Working Copy.................................. B1
C Project Proposal for a Hospital C1
D Sample Letter of Intent D1
E Sample Formal Contract for On-Site Consulting/Continuing Education E1
F Sample Subcontract F1

Index 269

I ENTREPRENEURSHIP

We want to draw you into the world of entrepreneurship and help you envision yourself in that role. In these first three chapters, we will describe how entrepreneurs operate, what they are like as people, and how they discover or create business opportunities. At a more personal level, we will show you how a nurse can use the experiences of other nurse entrepreneurs to find a niche in the marketplace and start a nurse-run business. Turn the page, and begin the journey.

1 ENTREPRENEURIAL ROLES

Today, *entrepreneur* is a status word. The proliferation of books and courses on the topic barely keeps pace with the dramatic rise in the number of people of diverse talents and backgrounds who are joining the entrepreneurial ranks. Nurses too are beginning to explore this option, though at a slower pace. If you are one of those nurses who have considered the possibility of an independent role, you probably have questions about what entrepreneuring entails and whether it would be a wise career move for you.

In this chapter, we develop a framework for assessing the personal benefits of an entrepreneurial career that can help you answer those questions. The key components of this framework are

1. an examination of the essential nature of entrepreneurs,
2. a review of the current socioeconomic and health-care trends that favor nurse entrepreneurs,
3. an analysis of the advantages and disadvantages of entrepreneurial roles, and
4. examples of the varied businesses nurse entrepreneurs have established.

DEFINITIONS

The entrepreneurial literature contains a variety of definitions of the role, each with its own specialty focus. For example, Church (1984) defines entrepreneurs solely from a business perspective, as "people who plan, organize, finance, and operate their own business" (p. 1). Although it is true that most entrepreneurs engage in these activities, we see this as a limited description of a complex role. Kirzner (1979) goes beyond this business orientation to underscore the innovative spirit of entrepreneurs, describing them as "alert . . . continually receptive to opportunities" (p. 7). He also points out that there is a substantial knowledge component to the entrepreneurial role: "entrepreneurial knowledge is a rarified abstract type of knowledge—the knowledge of where to obtain information (or other resources) and how to deploy it" (p. 8). Drucker (1985) highlights the creative essence of the role by defining the entrepreneur as one who "always searches for change, responds to it and explores it as an opportunity" (p. 28). Gilder (1984) considers entrepreneurs as part of the economic forces within a system and views them as individuals who "generate entirely new markets or theories" (p. 145).

Each of these authors examines a particular facet of the role, but none of them describes it completely. For this reason, we have formulated our own definition of the entrepreneur, one that reflects a broader conception of the role: an individual who assumes the total responsibility and risk for discovering or creating unique opportunities to use personal talents, skills, and energy, and who employs a strategic planning process to transform that opportunity into a marketable service or product. This definition takes into account the innovation, drive, foresight, and management that entrepreneurship demands, as well as the creative fertility and continual hard work that are essential for success. It also supports our belief that entrepreneurs are not an elite group but an assortment of more or less ordinary individuals whose common characteristic is their willingness to invest in and give of themselves to realize their goals. Nurses have the capacity to become entrepreneurs; and in fact the current environment, in health care and in society as a whole, is extremely favorable to such a career move.

TRENDS AFFECTING ENTREPRENEURIAL ROLES

The entrepreneurial spirit is part of the history of the United States. Individual enterprise expanded the frontiers, and small businesses made up the majority of the work economy in the early 1900s. Creative entrepreneurs flourished even in difficult times such as the depression of the 1930s or the big business era of the 1950s. Since the 1970s, entrepreneurial activity has accelerated, fueled by a variety of socioeconomic and health care–related changes. Change provides the impetus for innovation, and an examination of current societal trends confirms that the climate is now favorable for nurse entrepreneurs. The socioeconomic and health-care trends discussed in this section affect the entrepreneur in two ways: (1) by providing support (money, approval, or other resources) for new venture development, or (2) by generating new market opportunities.

Socioeconomic Trends

The socioeconomic forces relevant to entrepreneurs include

- a proentrepreneurial economy,
- a corporate focus on entrepreneurship,
- greater availability of educational and informational support,
- the growing prominence of women's issues, and
- an increasingly information-based society.

Proentrepreneurial Economy. The proentrepreneurial economy is the culmination of several interrelated developments, among which are (1) loss of confidence in established institutions—business, government, education, and medicine—with a concomitant increase in self-reliance, (2) a weak job market, and (3) greater diversity in the roles open to women.

Disillusionment and loss of confidence in traditional institutions was largely the result of the failure of these institutions to solve the problems facing them. Even when they did find solutions, it sometimes seemed that the solutions exacted too high a price in loss of freedom, mediocrity, and regimentation—consequences that outweighed the supposed benefits of the solutions. R. Mimi Clark Secor, of Nurse Practitioner Associates, designed her entrepreneurial role to overcome the aspects of a traditional role that were most problematic to her.

> I realized that I could best work in a setting that was supportive of my needs as an employee, and that just wasn't possible working under the thumb of a large organization, or even in partnership with other providers. So I did a little homework and plunged in.

Institutional failures, the widespread perception of those failures, and the unacceptability of the institutional solutions that were offered generated a movement toward greater self-reliance and a renewed sense that personal responsibility was the foundation of problem resolution. Increased interest in entrepreneurship was a natural result of greater self-reliance.

Nurses, too, have felt disillusionment with traditional systems. When asked to explain their decision to become entrepreneurs, many nurses responded in much the same way as Penny Hamlin, of Nurses Edu-Care/Resource Network.

> The single most significant factor in deciding to go into business was simply frustration with the traditional systems and a desire on both our

> parts to do *something* about it. I started teaching childbirth classes in 1971, and from that experience learned that a nurse can function very happily outside traditional settings. I was frustrated with the slow changes taking place in hospital/nursing homes and the general unwillingness to try new approaches. I was always too independent to fit in with the status quo or to settle into a daily routine.

For other nurses, the main source of frustration with traditional systems was inadequate care provided to patients/clients, as it was for Lenore Boles, of the Nurse Counseling Group.

> As a clinical instructor at a state hospital, I despaired at the care given clients and felt they needed another source of help. I originally saw us as helping chronically mentally ill clients.

The weak job market is the result of technologic changes, the move from an industrial base to a high-tech/information base, and the tremendous number of baby boomers seeking jobs. Some workers were permanently displaced from their high-paying jobs in the declining industries; others realized that the influx of baby boomers meant limited opportunities for success as it is usually defined in US society (working for someone else and climbing the corporate ladder). Still other workers in corporations and institutions retained their jobs and even attained some measure of success, but became frustrated. The institutions offered benefits, but these benefits were acquired at too high a cost in terms of personal freedom and creativity. For all these reasons, the time was ripe for the entrepreneurial explosion.

Women had additional incentives to become entrepreneurs, among them greater diversity in career options. Today, only one of seven American families fits the traditional definition of the nuclear family, in which the husband works and the wife stays home cooking, cleaning, and caring for the children (Naisbitt, 1984, p. 261). Nevertheless, even though more women are working outside the home, the major responsibility for child rearing and homemaking is still assigned to women. This, along with the realities of outside employment—lower wages for the same work, less opportunity for advancement, and lack of adequate support systems (such as child care)—has encouraged women to turn to entrepreneurship as a means of integrating all their actual or anticipated roles, earning a decent wage, and enjoying success on their own terms (Ballas & Hollas, 1984). For Carole Meola, of Management and Career Resources, limited opportunity was a major stumbling block: "There was no more upward mobility in the area I wanted or was qualified for—I was a victim of the 'plateau trap.' " For Dr. Dianne Moore, of Mooreinfo Inc., one of the main advantages of her home-based medical information service was that it gave her the "ability to interact with family easily when needed." These reasons could be cited by any potential entrepreneur, but they have a special significance for women.

By 1974, Baty could accurately state that "at no time and no place on earth have the conditions been more propitious for starting a new venture" (p. 8). This favorable climate is due not only to the factors already described but also to the general expectation that entrepreneurship will improve the economic base by creating new products, new jobs, and new wealth. Thanks to heightened awareness of the economic significance of entrepreneurial activities, venture capital for small businesses is more readily available now than in the past (Drucker, 1984, p. 58). Those small businesses that are likely to generate the greatest number of jobs tend to receive the most attention, but sole proprietorship enterprises reap the benefits of the renewed interest in entrepreneurship as well.

Of special importance for nurses are the areas in which these new businesses are being started. One third of the new ventures are in high-tech fields, and the remaining two thirds are divided among service, education and training, health care, and information. Women entrepreneurs are fueling the booming growth of the service economy: 40 percent of their businesses are in this sector, which provides 74 percent of US jobs ("1986," 1986, p. 35). Therefore, those business ventures that are most likely to attract nurse entrepreneurs are among those that have the best prospects for economic growth. This, coupled with the increased availability of venture capital, modifies the initial risk involved in starting most business.

Corporate Focus on Entrepreneurship. Corporations are beginning to recognize the relationship between entrepreneurial roles and survival in competitive markets. Naisbitt (1984) predicts that "we will restructure our businesses into smaller and smaller units, more entrepreneurial units, more participatory units" (p. 17). Deal and Kennedy (1982) characterize the decentralized corporation of the future as "the atomized organization which will liberate people to the degree of entrepreneurship they want and can handle" (p. 186). Drucker (1985) states emphatically that "today's businesses, especially the large ones, simply will not survive in this period of rapid change and innovation unless they acquire entrepreneurial competence" (p. 14). He further concludes that it is public institutions, such as hospitals, that face the greatest pressure to be entrepreneurial in order to survive.

This changing corporate emphasis has three potential benefits. First, corporations will be conditioned to make use of entrepreneurial expertise and will be a receptive market for the external specialty consultant. Second, there will be an increased demand for consultants who can develop the entrepreneurial skills of employees and help organizations alter their policies and cultures in order to stimulate and support innovation. Third, those nurses who decide that the risks of independence outweigh the benefits will be more likely to find corporate cultures in which their entrepreneurial spirit can thrive.

Educational and Informational Support. Educational institutions have kept pace with economic and corporate developments and have strengthened their emphasis on entrepreneurship in both graduate and undergraduate programs (Shomes, 1986, p. 84). Universities and junior colleges now include courses on small business development and management in their continuing education programs. Small business associations, women's groups, and professional nurses' associations sponsor seminars and disseminate literature on entrepreneurship. As the number of nurse entrepreneurs increases, their networks for support and information are strengthened. These expanding information networks are a valuable resource for developing individual competencies, finding peer support, and minimizing the potential errors a new nurse entrepreneur is likely to make.

The Nurse Consultants Association (414 Plaza Drive, Suite 209, Westmont, Illinois 60559) is an example of an organization that provides a network for nurse entrepreneurs. Its purposes are to establish a nurse consultants' network, formulate a method of promoting quality nurse consulting services, and provide a vehicle through which consultants' continued learning needs can be met. To be considered for membership, applicants must

- be currently licensed as a registered nurse,
- be working as a nurse consultant,
- not be involved in direct patient care while holding this position,
- receive at least 60 percent of their annual income from or spend at least 60 percent of their time in this position,
- give evidence of education and experience at a level appropriate for the area of consultation, and
- be self-employed or work for a health care–related business or industry.

Women's Issues. Some nurses are men, but the great majority are women. Accordingly, the efforts of groups seeking to enhance the rights and status of women have have a considerable effect on the career options open to nurses. Alternatives to women's traditional roles have indeed been developed, but there is still a great deal of confusion about how these roles mesh with what is traditionally expected of women. Women are faced with a typical transitional situation, in which society expects that they continue to fulfill their traditional roles while developing their new identity.

The expectation that women retain the primary responsibility for homemaking and child rearing affects the credibility of women on the job and perpetuates the cycle of inadequate support systems, low pay, and lack of equal advancement opportunities. Women's loyalties, professionalism, and commitment to the business world are viewed as being less than total, and probably temporary. A recent study dramatically documents that women maintain the majority of child-rearing and homemaking responsibilities. Eighty-two percent of the women surveyed did all or most of the housework. Employed wives spent an average of 26 hours per week on housework, while their husbands spent an average of 36 minutes per week (Cruver, 1986, p. 5D). If you are uncertain about where you fit into this analysis, use Exercise 1.1 to estimate the amount of noncareer work that you routinely perform.

✔ Exercise 1.1 Noncareer Work of Working Women.

If you do not live alone, the chances are high that you assume some housework and family responsibilities with or for a significant other in addition to your work outside the home.

Instructions. In the left column, indicate the percent of the time that you perform each activity listed; in the right, indicate the percent of the time that someone living with you performs it. For example, if you share the task of making dinner equally with your spouse, write "50 percent" for that activity in both columns.

Activity		Percent of Time You Do	Percent of Time Others Do
1. Put away personal belongings	Your own		
	Others'		
2. Dust			
3. Vacuum			
4. Sweep or mop floors			
5. Make beds			
6. Change sheets			
7. Hang up wet towels after shower			
8. Clean bathroom			
9. Clean up after between-meal snacks			
10. Cook meals			
11. Set table			
12. Do dishes and put them away			
13. Do laundry			

Activity	Percent of Time You Do	Percent of Time Others Do
14. Hang up clothes		
15. Clean out pockets and turn socks and clothes right side out before putting them in laundry		
16. Iron		
17. Take out garbage		
18. Fix/mend broken things around house		
19. Run errands		
20. Drive others to appointments, programs, etc.		
21. Pack suitcases for a trip		
22. Unpack after a trip		
23. Do yard work		
24. Wash windows		
25. Take car for repairs		
26. Pay bills		
27. Provide personal care (bathing, combing hair, dressing) for another		
28. Shop for groceries		

Scoring. For each score of 50 percent or less in your column, give yourself 1 point.

If your score was 0 to 7, maybe you are trying too hard. Take an assertiveness course and start setting firm limits on how much you will do. Learn to negotiate and delegate.

If your score was 8 to 15, you are doing better, but you probably still feel exhausted most of the time. Start delegating more.

If your score was 16 to 22, you are getting good at negotiating and delegating. Hone your skills and ask for more equal time sharing.

If your score was 23 to 28, you are on the right track. You probably have the good time utilization and delegation skills that entrepreneurs need.

Adapted from Cruver (1986). Used with permission.

In an effort to cope with the realities of their personal and professional existence, women have sought strategies that will permit them to bring some flexibility, control, and balance to their lives. For many women, entrepreneurship is more than a career strategy: It is a life strategy that permits them to develop their capacity to fill strategy that permits them to develop their capacity to fill a wide variety of possible roles (Nobel, 1986, p. 46). Three times as many women are starting businesses as men. Women own more then 25 percent of sole proprietorship businesses (Wojahn, 1986, p. 46). There are 3 million female entrepreneurs in the United States, and women-owned businesses increased at a rate of 6.9 percent per year between 1977 and 1982 ("Women Entrepreneurs," 1986, p. 33).

The future of women entrepreneurs has never looked brighter. Some see entrepreneurship as the mechanism that will permit women to attain full equality in employment. "Once there are a sufficient number of women running their own businesses, the corporate barriers could begin to lift" (Connelly, 1986, p. 5A).

The Information Society. The information explosion keeps us running a frantic race to avoid obsolescence. As Naisbitt (1984) remarks, "we are drowning in information but starved for knowledge" (p. 17). The computer has not only altered the way in which we process information but also accelerated the pace of information exchange and created a pervasive sense of information overload.

These very dilemmas create entrepreneurial opportunities. An obvious example is the expanding market for persons with computer expertise. A more important one, however, is the growing critical demand for the knowledge expert described by Kirzner (1979, p. 8). Knowledge workers who can identify what knowledge is needed by whom and retrieve that information rapidly will discover that myriad opportunities are open to them. Nurses are knowledge experts of just this type, and they have a broad range of potential clients, including patients, families, other health care workers, health care agencies, and health information consumers (such as lawyers).

Dr. Carolyn Brose and Dr. Norma Lewis are partners in two corporations, Andicore and Nu Vision. Both companies are based on recognition of the opportunities afforded to nurses by the computer and information explosions. Dr. Brose describes Nu Vision as a technology-based educational support materials company that also assists clients (usually schools of nursing) in using the computer to develop curricula, course work, and a systems approach to education. The stimulus for the business was the desire to be on the cutting edge of the computerization of nursing and nursing education. Dr. Lewis describes Andicore's service as health education using interactive video technology. Employers of health care providers, such as physicians, nurses, paramedics, police officers and firefighters, are Andicore's clients. The company offers consultation to assess learning needs, provides interactive video equipment to help learners maintain and develop psychomotor skills (e.g., CPR), and develops courseware for the interactive learning system. This courseware has included examples of material on electronic fetal heart monitoring, physical assessment, and advanced cardiac life support for the paramedic.

Nursing and Health Care Trends

Consideration of the numerous complex changes now taking place in nursing and health care reveals five major trends that can have an impact on the climate for nurse entrepreneurs.

- the empowerment of nursing,
- the high tech–high touch connection,
- movement of patients with high-acuity needs to nontraditional settings,
- increased consumer awareness, and
- the restructuring of health-care provider organizations.

Empowerment of Nursing. Nursing has made significant progress toward being recognized as a profession capable of and entitled to self-determination. Emphasis on nursing diagnosis and practice-related research has highlighted nurses' unique role in helping clients identify and resolve health-related problems. Nursing's emphasis on the total person extends the boundaries of nursing practice beyond the limits of medicine, and the outcomes of recent litigation support this expansion of boundaries. R. Mimi Clarke Secor of Nurse Practitioner Associates expresses sentiments that are representative:

> I decided, even though there were many health settings and providers in the Boston area providing women's health care, that there was a crying need for services delivered in a uniquely warm, supportive manner.

Nancy Dirubbo, of Laconia Women's Health Center, also set up a center to bring nursing's special brand of care to her patients.

> Women sought GYN care through providers 30 to 40 miles away because they did not like the medical-model MD group GYN practice in our town. Most traveled to see nurse practitioners or certified nurse midwives. I wanted to offer that kind of service locally. My nursing focus versus the strict medical model is what patients seem to want. I listen and spend time with clients—visits average 20 minutes, versus

> the average MD visit time of seven minutes. I also have more availability and accessibility: when patients call I get back to them, usually within one or two hours.

As nurses continue to demonstrate that they can provide high-quality, cost-effective solutions to health care problems, third-party payors are increasingly being persuaded to reimburse nurse providers directly. The experience of Jamie Hills, of New Care Concepts Inc., illustrates this point.

> In 1982, federal funds became available to families with chronically ill or disabled children who require long-term hospitalization to provide for care at home. New Care Concepts was founded on the premise that quality, comprehensive, cost-effective home health care is a viable alternative to long-term hospitalization.
>
> In comparing the costs of hospitalization to the cost of having New Care Concepts provide care for the child at home, a monthly savings of about 33 percent was realized. Reimbursement for New Care Concepts services is provided by both the federal government and private insurance companies.

Nurses have pursued other avenues to power and influence as well. Nurse administrators have successfully assumed corporate responsibilities in health care organizations, becoming essential members of strategic planning teams. At the national level, nurses are acquiring political savvy and using it to influence major policy decisions for nursing and health care. Nurse-run businesses are on the rise, setting the precedent for independent practice. Many nurses believe that owning their own professional for-profit corporations is also the key to changing nursing employment practices and nursing itself. This major shift in the marketing of nursing services promises to lead to the achievement of a truly professional status (Milhaven, 1984, p. 48).

In short, nurses are acquiring the critical competencies necessary for successful entrepreneurship and consulting. As a result, aspiring nurse entrepreneurs will find it easier to be accepted, to discover available markets, to obtain reimbursement for their services, and generally to be successful in business.

High Tech–High Touch. As the technologic approaches to diagnosis and treatment multiply and become more complex, demand for nursing expertise grows in three ways. First, clients surrounded by this confusing and sometimes frightening technology need some kind of human-oriented support if they are to understand it and adapt to the lifestyle changes it creates. Nursing expertise can provide this support. Second, the technology generates new information. The person best qualified to answer questions about how to gather this information, how to assess its impact, and how to disseminate it so that clients' needs are met in the most effective way is the provider closest to the client, namely, the nurse. Third, technologic advances foster specialization and create a demand for new skills. Many health care providers will find themselves needing to "retool" periodically in order to stay up to date. The nurse entrepreneur with specialized expertise and teaching-learning skills can meet this challenge.

Increased Patient Acuity in Nonacute Settings. Because of strict admission criteria and patterns of early discharge, there is a growing tendency to transfer patients with high-acuity illness needs from hospitals to community and extended care facilities. Anne Butts, of Nurse Care Limited, had the opportunity, as a hospital employee, to observe the effect of early patient discharges at first hand.

> I saw an influx of discharged patients [returning to the hospital] due to poor discharge planning and follow-up, and poor quality local home health-care services. Nurse Care Limited provides home care for patients requiring IV therapy.

The effects of early discharge on patients, families, and caregivers have been the stretching of available resources, knowledge deficits, and a proliferation of new but not necessarily qualified provider systems. The experience of being a caregiver to a family member at home was the impetus for Dr. Barbara Bohny's corporation, New Hope Respite and Home Care.

> I cared for my mother at home for eight years. She was a stroke victim. I became aware of the lack of services for people trying to care for someone at home. Respite care, a desperately needed service, was not available. There were no respite care services available in the state of New Jersey at the time I began this service. New Hope provides both home nursing care and relief for family members from caregiving responsibilities.

Clients search for information about how to care for themselves or their families, where to obtain monetary or other resources, how to work through the maze of reimbursement forms and bureaucratic structures, and how to assess the quality of care they are given in order to make informed health care choices. Caregivers for their part, need to develop new skills, update acuity data systems, and address the changes now occurring through creative problem solving. The changes in the system are so at odds with the expectations and values of the recent past that the opportunities for nursing innovation are numerous.

Increased Consumer Awareness. As regards health care, consumers are now more cost-conscious, quality-conscious, and wellness-oriented than ever before. They are anxious to keep up with health care trends so that they can make informed decisions for themselves. The wellness phenomenon provides an ideal environment for the development of nurse-run clinics in which advanced nursing practice skills are used in client-centered wellness care. Dianne Duchesne, executive director of Nurses in Transition, has taken the wellness concept a step further. Her business helps nurses gain and give support in using wellness concepts in their practices.

> Our purpose is to enhance the personal professional healing potential of nurses. We do this by
>
> - exploring the wide variety of healing approaches and creative educational processes,
> - creating an environment supportive to the birth and growth of nurses' visions, and
> - encouraging nurses to love and accept each other unconditionally.
>
> The nurses who are attracted to Nurses in Transition have a vision which includes wellness orientation, collaborative approaches to health and healing. Many come with a broad base of healing perspectives including ancient, conventional, and cross-cultural systems, They take every opportunity to encourage and educate clients to be active participants in the healing process. Support and acceptance is essential for nurses who are moving beyond traditional modes of practice and becoming powerful health catalysts. As members of Nurses in Transition, nurses educate one another and role model creative approaches to healing themselves and clients.

Restructuring of Health-Care Provider Organizations. Health-care institutions are in constant flux as they adapt to dramatic external pressures, downsizing, merging, or expanding into new markets. The number of new provider agencies has risen rapidly. For-profit hospitals have sharpened the competitive focus of traditional agencies and raised questions (as yet unanswered) about how they will affect health care in the nation as a whole. Many agencies are looking for ways of reducing staff, such as by purchasing expert services on a need basis. Staff members are moving from old work areas as census declines or changing work specialties in order to keep their jobs. Nurses are moving to the new agencies or into community and long-term care institutions as patient census increases in these settings. The nurse entrepreneur has many services to offer in this shifting scene. Two examples are

- team-building consultation as staff members move to a new area in an agency or as new agencies start up and
- providing a needed service to multiple agencies (e.g., staff development, computer expertise, and patient education) as an independent supplier.

Joan Nelson, of Nelson Institute, is one nurse who serves multiple agencies as an independent supplier of an essential service:

> Nelson Institute provides outpatient alcohol/drug assessment and counseling services to patients who are referred by numerous community organizations. A partial list of referral sources includes the State Division of Vocational Rehabilitation, judges, child protection agencies, and physicians. I started in this business because alcohol/drug abuse are our number one health problem, and the needs were not being addressed. I like the work and keep improving the services. The assessment tool I constructed and designed in the best I've seen. My program design results in a high recovery rate.

Two other services nurse entrepreneurs can offer are

- developing quality assurance programs for new organizations
- patient and family counseling and education for clients in a variety of agencies.

Drucker (1985) writes that successful innovators "exploit change" (p. 35). In this section, we have examined selected changes and the opportunities they created for nurse entrepreneurs. These examples of nurse-run businesses illustrate how current trends favor your entrepreneurial endeavors. Even a favorable trend analysis, however, must be evaluated in relation to the overall advantages and disadvantages for the individual anticipating an entrepreneurial career move.

ADVANTAGES AND DISADVANTAGES

As we compare our personal experiences with those of the nurse entrepreneurs who contributed to this book, we find that we note many of the same advantages and disadvantages. The overview in Table 1.1 represents a composite of these shared experiences and strategies. We list advantages both to encourage you and to stimulate you to think about the unique benefits entrepreneurship might offer you. We identify disadvantages not as deterrents but as problems that can be minimized or eliminated by means of strategic planning.

It is important for you, as a potential entrepreneur, to identify which of the advantages and disadvantages listed in Table 1.1 apply to your situation. Once you establish a clear idea of the risks you might encounter, you can develop a strategic plan to minimize the chance of failure.

There is a myth that entrepreneurs take tremendous risks. Although successful entrepreneurs are risk takers, McClelland (1961) points out that they

TABLE 1.1 Strategies for Maximizing Advantages and Minimizing Disadvantages of Entrepreneurial Role

Entrepreneurial Characteristic	Advantages	Disadvantages	Strategies
Freedom Flexibility	You can focus your energies on work that interests you.	The market for services you enjoy providing may dry up.	Apply strategic planning concepts to stay ahead of market needs.
	You can choose the time and place for work.	Workload varies, with periods of high volume alternating with low-volume periods.	Establish clear goals and review them daily. Plan activities for down time (writing an article, taking a course.
	You can balance a variety of roles more easily.	It can become difficult to separate personal and work time or limit interruptions, especially if you are working at home.	Develop time management skills early. Structure consistent worktime periods. Make sure you have a separate workspace if you work at home.
	Because you work in a variety of settings, your perspective is broadened to a "big picture" of nursing and health care issues.		Be ready to change and learn new skills to match new market demands. Stay current with professional issues.

(continued)

TABLE 1.1 Strategies for Maximizing Advantages and Minimizing Disadvantages of Entrepreneurial Role

Entrepreneurial Characteristic	Advantages	Disadvantages	Strategies
Independence	You are free to structure your approach to a particular project or problem.	You suffer from loneliness or self-doubt. You lack a peer group.	Keep active in professional organizations. Establish networks with other entrepreneurs, especially women entrepreneurs.
	You can assume total responsibility for the quality and outcome of projects.	You lack support and understanding from significant others (this is especially true for women).	Find a mentor.
Control of reimbursement	You can identify and charge fees appropriate to your skills and amount of work	Nurses tend to underprice themselves.	Make sure you establish a price structure that is equitable.
	You can take advantage of opportunities to increase your income.	You are prey to financial uncertainty. You may experience decreased income or at least inconsistent income because of variable work opportunities.	Prepare for possible decrease in income by having at least 6 months to 1 year of backup resources. Start up your entrepreneurial activity on a part-time basis until your income reaches an appropriate level.

(continued)

TABLE 1.1 Strategies for Maximizing Advantages and Minimizing Disadvantages of Entrepreneurial Role

Entrepreneurial Characteristic	Advantages	Disadvantages	Strategies
Challenge and Growth	New opportunities and requests for services stimulate growth and make you set stretching goals.	As new areas of need develop, they create requests for your services that demand new knowledge and skills from you.	Keep an eye on market trends so you know what needs are being created. Maintain expertise in your field via reading, workshops, and profesional associations.
Enhanced problem solving	You can apply your problem-solving skills to facilitate change in others. As an external consultant, you can discern and describe problems, recognize institutional norms that perpetuate them, and suggest remedies that can be implemented within the culture.	Clients may have a hidden agenda.	Develop a contract with outcome criteria and mutual expectations clearly defined.
		Your ability to appropriately identify destructive group norms may be limited.	Develop expertise in diagnosis of group and organizational processes.
		Conflict situations may arise because of your interventions.	Use constructive confrontation approaches to resolve conflicts.
		Your suggestions may be ignored.	Establish problem ownership and recognize that the client is free to ignore your advice. Build implementation strategies and support mechanisms into your change plan so that suggestions can be implemented appropriately.

(continued)

TABLE 1.1 Strategies for Maximizing Advantages and Minimizing Disadvantages of Entrepreneurial Role

Entrepreneurial Characteristic	Advantages	Disadvantages	Strategies
Altered self-esteem	Creating an independent and profitable practice results in enhanced self-confidence and self-esteem that is unparalleled in most jobs.	The failure or rejection of a project or proposal damages your self-esteem. The ultimate failure of the business may have an adverse effect on your self-confidence.	View failures in a business rather than a personal context. Learn from the failure and use these lessons to create the next success. Even if the business fails, you will have learned new skills and grown professionally.

"blossom under conditions of moderate uncertainty where their efforts or skill can make a difference in the outcome" (p. 211). For this reason, successful entrepreneurs use risk analysis to avoid being at the mercy of luck or chance. Entrepreneurs are planners rather than gamblers: the entrepreneurial role entails *moderate* risk taking controlled by competent analysis and planning.

We began that process of analysis and planning by examining the nature of the entrepreneurial role, the trends supportive of nurses as entrepreneurs, and the comparative advantages and disadvantages of the role while presenting strategies to handle potential risks. Before proceeding to chapter 2, complete Exercise 1.2, and use the framework developed in this chapter to decide if you can meet your personal and professional goals as an entrepreneur.

✔ Exercise 1.2 Entrepreneurial Career Decision Making.

1. What aspects of the entrepreneurial role most appeal to you?

   Personally:

   Professionally:

2. What trends do you see that support your entrepreneurial efforts?

3. What do you see as the advantages and disadvantages of the entrepreneurial role, and what strategies would you employ to overcome the disadvantages?

Advantages	Disadvantages	Strategies

4. On a scale of 0 to 10, how would you rate your attraction to the entrepreneurial role? (Circle the appropriate number.)

0	1	2	3	4	5	6	7	8	9	10
It's not for me.										I'm sold on the idea; I want to learn more.

Now that you have evaluated your personal attraction to an entrepreneurial career, you are ready to learn more about what characteristics entrepreneurs possess and how to develop your entrepreneurial opportunities into marketable ideas. The next two chapters will help you do this.

2 CHARACTERISTICS OF SUCCESSFUL ENTREPRENEURS

ENTREPRENEURS' CAREER PATH

Step 1: Viable Options

People who become entrepreneurs follow a surprisingly consistent path toward achieving that status (Welsh & White, 1983, pp. 57–63). The first step in the journey is to make the decision that entrepreneuring is a viable career option. This decision can be made for a variety of reasons: a role model, someone with a similar background, may start a successful business; or an individual may have an intrinsic belief in his or her ability to be an independent spirit. Carolyn Edison, of Family Health Care, Inc., exemplifies such an "I can do it" spirit.

> I graduated from nursing school in 1974 and was encouraged to be visionary and assertive. In fact, my entire life has pointed in that direction. I always believed I could do anything I wanted, and nursing seemed a good way to do just that. I believe the public should have direct access to nurses and that nurses should be paid directly, not through a physician. That belief led me to start my own business in 1977 providing education, assessment, and referral to families to help them reach a high level of wellness. Currently, I limit my practice to well-child conferences and work with juvenile offenders. Private practice provides me with autonomy, personal satisfaction, and the capacity for unlimited income. My advice for the potential nurse entrepreneur is GO FOR IT. There is no magic formula; just do it.

In some cases, an idea for a viable business is discovered, an idea that is so terrific that the potential entrepreneur is simply unable to resist it. Sometimes, experiences at work provide the impetus to start a business. The opportunity to control and direct a significant project may be sufficient to allow the entrepreneur to conclude that he or she is indeed capable of favorably influencing the outcome of a project, and in fact enjoys this type of challenge and reward so much that it only makes sense to explore entrepreneurship. Geneie Everett Fellows, of Humanistic Programming and Planning, found such an irresistible opportunity through a work experience.

> I was involved in planning a new critical care wing while head nurse of a surgical intensive care/coronary care unit. After working with the architects for two years, I realized that nurses can make a difference if involved early enough. Since the inception of my business in 1983, I have provided facility planning, space planning, architectural planning, postoccupancy evaluation, and equipment planning consultation. I emphasize a user/people involvement in the planning process with a focus on the humanistic needs to be incorporated in a building. My business has given me flexibility, independence, and a sense of pride in my success.

Step 2: Gathering Information

The second step in the entrepreneur's career path is to obtain more information about the product or service that will form the basis of the business. This knowledge is gained from a close relationship to the consumer (see Chapter 3). From this vantage point, the entrepreneur identifies gaps or problems—e.g., poor quality, sloppy service, or lack of information—that may become the crux of the business concept.

Step 3: Developing the Concept

The third step is to develop a business concept. After identifying the gaps that exist in current products or services, the entrepreneur plans the methodology that will permit him or her to compete with existing companies. The business concept addresses some need in that customer that either has not been met or has been poorly met.

Entrepreneurs typically move back and forth between steps 2 and 3. More information is obtained, and the business concept is adjusted, changed, or reaffirmed accordingly. It is not until a traumatic event occurs that the entrepreneur actually puts the plan into action.

Step 4: Traumatic Event

The fourth step is the occurrence of a traumatic event. This event is often the impetus for a change from a career as an employee to an entrepreneurial career. The traumatic event differs from one entrepreneur to the next. For some, it is a specific event, such as quitting a job just prior to getting fired, getting fired, a watershed birthday (30, 40, 50), a divorce, or the birth of a child. For others, it is more of a cumulative condition: boredom with the job, intense resentment at taking orders, a hunger for success left unfulfilled by the job, or a pervasive anxiety that life is passing you by (Cook, 1986, p. 10).

Whatever the traumatic event, it is significant in that it causes the individual to decide, once and for all, to take matters into his or her own hands at any cost (Aldrich, 1986, p. 65). Carol Haller, of Haller's Nursing Care, Inc., went through this developmental process before her 1980 business start-up.

> The idea first came to me as an RN student working on my BSN. I attended a lecture by Lucille Kinlein and liked the idea of being independent. My personal experience caring for my terminally ill father pointed out the need for nurses to be available to clients without a physician referral. After my father's death, I was not employed and wanted a job that met all my requirements. Since that kind of job didn't exist, I started out in private practice nursing and then started the registry when I repeatedly saw a need for this service. My business provides home nursing care and hospital sitters on a 24-hour basis. I strive to provide personal, caring service to meet the individual needs of each client and worker. My motto and business philosophy is "nursing care by nurses who care." From the original idea, a business has developed that allows me to control my own destiny and gives me the convenience and flexibility that are important to me.

Step 5: Testing

The fifth step is to make the business concept work once. The entrepreneur does whatever must be done, seizing any opportunity to convince that first customer that this produce or service is superior. Marcia Harris, of Home Hospice Nursing, Inc., is someone who kept on going after that first successful client contact.

> There were three stimuli for our business idea: the hospice movement itself, dissatisfaction with the quality of home nursing services for extended hours of bedside care, and the lack of professionals in our area who were skilled in home management of the physical and psychosocial needs of terminally ill patients and families. After hemming and hawing for months about whether or not to commit ourselves, a local clergyman provided the shot in the arm we needed. A member of his congregation needed our services; he convinced us; we started and kept on going. We have developed a practice that is unique because all our services are in-house and provided by our trained staff, not farmed out to other agencies. We provide our clients with a 24-hour presence. That first client experience resulted in the 1980 start-up of what is today a highly successful nurse-run business. If you are creative, gutsy, and dissatisfied in your current role, go for it! With a lot of preplanning and thought, you could have little to lose and everything to gain.

Step 6: Growth

The sixth step is to perceive growth opportunities. These opportunities present themselves in various ways. One is adding to the number and types of services or products provided; another is franchising the business. Each new option makes it necessary for the entrepreneur to evaluate the opportunity by returning to earlier steps: gaining product and market knowledge, developing a business concept, and making the concept work once. Since she began her business in 1972, Edna A. Lauterbach, of Health Savers, Inc., has expanded her business as new, and sometimes unexpected, client demands emerged.

> I hung a sign and placed ads for home care and immediately received requests for private duty in the hospital. I met that need, and then received requests for hospital staffing. I met that need while working to change home care legislation. I'm now meeting the need for home care. Health Savers, Inc., provides certified home health care, staffing, and educational programs to a broad client base. Clients include private patients, insurance companies, state agencies, hospitals, nursing homes, schools, and prisons. A willingness to take risks, determination, and a blind passion for what I do are the strengths that I bring to the business and its growth.

Step 7: Expansion

The seventh and last step in the entrepreneur's career path is to expand significantly. It is usually at this point that the business requires an organizational structure, employees, policies, and procedures. The entrepreneur may, however, be unable to run the business because of his or her particular inherent combination of entrepreneurial characteristics. Some entrepreneurs choose to sell the business; others change sufficiently to handle the required tasks; and still others acquire a management team to handle the aspects that are difficult for them. Some entrepreneurs continually repeat this process, selling the successful business so that they can return to repeat those activities that are most suited to their temperament and strengths. That temperament and those strengths make up the entrepreneurial personality described in the next section.

THE ENTREPRENEURIAL PERSONALITY

Successful entrepreneurs share numerous personal characteristics. Among these characteristics are

- willingness to take moderate risks,
- self-confidence and an internal locus of control,
- determination and perseverance,

- interpersonal skills,
- low need for status,
- comprehensive awareness,
- need to control and direct,
- physical and mental resiliency, and
- a need for achievement.

Risk Taking

Entrepreneurs are often characterized as individuals who assume tremendous risks. In reality, however, they prefer moderate risks: ones that are challenging but can be favorably influenced by skill and judgment. Before assuming risks of even moderate intensity, entrepreneurs clearly and carefully consider every pertinent aspect. It is not until they are completely convinced that the risk is manageable and the outcome predictable that they will commit themselves to a project. Once committed, however, they plow through with astounding determination and perseverance until they reach their goals. Linda Hackett took this kind of calculated risk in 1978, when she and Lenore Boles started their own psychotherapy and counseling practice, Nurse Counseling Group.

> I was the clinical specialist on an inpatient psychiatric unit, and Lenore Boles was an instructor with students on the unit. We felt we could deliver better psychiatric care to clients, and we believed that clients deserved an alternative source of health care. There were no other nurses in private practice in our area at the time; we were both part of the Mental Health Community and knew the market. These observations convinced us, and we decided to go into business. Within one year, we paid our debts and were earning money. I have gained autonomy in client care, scheduling flexibility, satisfaction as a therapist, and a sense of achieving for nursing.

Self-Confidence and Internal Locus of Control

Self-confidence is a common entrepreneurial trait. Entrepreneurs believe in themselves, in their ideas, and in their course of action. They feel most self-confident when they are in control: anything is possible when they direct the project, but any loss of control (such as being a team member rather than the leader) results in loss of confidence, frustration, and anger. They place a high value on achievement, independence, and effective leadership.

Another common trait of entrepreneurs is intrinsic belief in their own ability to affect the outcomes of their endeavors; they are rarely fatalistic.

This internal locus of control is the springboard for many of the other characteristics listed. Barb Dalpez, who owns Moss Bay Preventive Medicine with her physician partner, possesses this kind of intrinsic belief in herself and her practice.

> I was forced to become an entrepreneur because I didn't seem to fit into the conventional environment. Alternative health care concepts, such as therapeutic touch and accupressure, aren't accepted in the hospital setting. I believe I have developed my ability to practice the art of nursing and am able to give my patients large doses of unconditional love and caring. I am trained in several alternative healing methods and am able to help heal on different levels: physical, emotional, and spiritual. I love nursing and I do it well. My personal strengths are:
>
> 1. self-esteem (I'm equal to anything; I assume I'll be a success!),
> 2. positive thinking (negative thoughts aren't part of my vocabulary),
> 3. a strong sense of spirituality (I trust when I ask for things; visual imagery is part of this—we are what we think).
>
> I mapped out this ideal job two years ago; my list had about 20 requirements. Every requirement was met, except that I'm earning more money than anticipated. I love all aspects of what I'm doing. I can be all I want to be.

Determination and Perseverance

Entrepreneurs know that their ideas are sound and that they will work. This thought alone sustains their confidence in the face of excruciating rejection, financial hardship, and an endless and varied array of setbacks.

After analyzing Thomas Edison and Henry Ford at first hand for many years, Napoleon Hill concluded, "I have found no quality, save persistence, in either of them that even remotely suggested the major source of their stupendous achievements" (Cook, 1986, p. 27). Andrea Karlin, executive director of Northwest Neighborhood Nurses, Inc., has pursued her ideal of a nurse-managed nonprofit clinic with similar zeal and determination.

> I was familiar with this area of Portland, Oregon, and the needs of elderly residents. Recent business experience convinced me that I would enjoy a business involving nursing and the elderly. I was positive that nurses were capable and should be contributing to the community. We provide nursing care primarily to low-income elderly, but we also respond to many telephone requests for care or information from people of all ages. We have no set fees; instead, we developed a schedule of suggested donations for services. People pay what they can. It is a unique opportunity to promote nursing as a valid and important component of

> health care. However, it is frustrating to have to keep explaining what nursing is and is not, to exist in a hand-to-mouth fashion while trying to find stable support; and it is cumbersome to work through a board of directors. Perseverance is one of my strenghts. I just keep trying; continuing to exist is an accomplishment.

Interpersonal Skills

Many entrepreneurs possess interpersonal skills to only a moderate degree. Under normal circumstances, this skill level is sufficient for the accomplishment of their goals in the early stages of building a business. In certain conditions, however, it tends to create problems for them.

When combined with a propensity to be more concerned about accomplishments than about people's feelings and a need to maintain control, moderate levels of interpersonal skills become problematic. For the entrepreneur whose business has grown sufficiently to require an organizational structure and employees, this combination of circumstances creates an environment in which employees resent the constant interference they encounter in trying to do their jobs, as well as the entrepreneur's apparent insensitivity to their feelings in bypassing organizational structure and lines of authority. Employees feel that their competence is being questioned; this leads to internal conflict, organizational instability, and constant employee turnover. Unless the entrepreneur's behavior changes, the business is destined to fail (Connelly, 1986, p. 27D).

Nurses have a major advantage in this area, in that they usually have developed the interpersonal and caring skills that make them effective in managing or collaborating with others. Sheila Felberbaum, of A Round The Clock Temporary Services, Inc., is a nurse entrepreneur whose combination of business and interpersonal skills has enhanced the overall quality of a growing business.

> In 1977, I was one of the first people to develop and run a home care agency. Our services are provided in the most professional manner possible. The care of people is reflected not only in the way patients are treated, but in the way staff are handled. I learned to hire people with skills different than mine, to appreciate other ways of working in order to complement my style, and to delegate (most difficult). As the business grew, I became more involved in administration and began to miss client contact. I learned to use therapeutic touch, imagery, and relaxation and began a small private practice in order to interact with clients again. That led me to obtain an MSW and expand my skills as a therapist. The combination of the ability to fight against obstacles, work hard, and love what I do *plus* care deeply about people and believe that others are intrinsically of great worth allows me to persevere when things seem difficult.

Low Need for Status

External evidence of success—big houses, expensive clothes, cars and money—are not important to the entrepreneur for the purpose of enhancing status. The external trappings are not there to impress others: they are there to provide an accounting system that allows the entrepreneur to keep track of how well he or she is doing by conventional standards. Achievement and successful functioning in the entrepreneurial mode meet the entrepreneur's status needs. Judy Dean, of Health Care Consultants of Wisconsin, describes the personal satisfaction that she and her partners find in entrepreneurship.

> Our business started in 1985. We provide educational services, primarily continuing education programs, to a variety of health care agencies. As a group of nursing faculty, we represent a broad specialty base and can tailor programs to meet the specific needs of a client. The main advantages have been the opportunity to be your own boss, being able to develop your own potential, and controlling your own income. There is also the personal and professional pride in the quality product produced. In addition, learning new skills like sales and marketing has opened new vistas for many of us.

Comprehensive Awareness

The number of tasks required to keep a small business operating is astronomical. While working at the task at hand, the entrepreneur must also maintain an awareness of the needs and direction of the business in general. The task at hand must be put into perspective and its value measured against the growth and survival of the operation as a whole. Alternative plans are generated every step of the way, and changes are implemented whenever they are needed to achieve overall business objectives. Alice Marie Kotkowski, president of AMK Associates, operates a multifocused business that depends upon continual perceptive assessment of the marketplace.

> AMK Associates is a health-care industry consulting firm providing new channels of distribution for health-care institutions, product manufacturers, and service companies while opening new vistas to nurses making a transition to a business environment. The range of services provided includes recruiting, training, brokering, and consulting. My unique background has allowed me to understand both sides of the health-care dollar, as well as the essence and realities of nursing. An entrepreneur must be open to new learning and opportunities to stay on top of the market. I attend a variety of programs and workshops and read textbooks and periodicals in a variety of subject areas. I joined several business and professional associations and became active on boards and committees. Networking is very important; women don't always understand

> this. In addition, I'm a workaholic. Entrepreneurs don't have 40-hour weeks. It's important to focus on long range planning and goals.

Success is a journey, not an immediate destination.

Need to Control and Direct

Entrepreneurs believe that they can accomplish their objectives best if they have total and complete control over what is to be done and how it is to be done. They do not do well in traditional organizations in which someone is in authority over them, or in circumstances that require them to ask permission, compromise, or be a part of a team. Dr. Candice Teles provides psychotherapy and wellness counseling to children and adults. Her feelings about the needs and rewards of independence are echoed by most of the nurse entrepreneurs in our survey.

> I have an entrepreneurial personality, and the bureaucracy of institutions generates a feeling of suffocation and alienation in me. I like freedom, autonomy, and I want to make a decent income. A nurse mentor who has a nutrition practice provided the catalyst for me to start a business of my own. When I finally had an office with many windows, wonderful furniture, and clients, it shocked me to realize how easy it is to get what we deserve. I have gained autonomy, independence, increased meaning, and increased earnings.

Physical and Mental Resiliency

Entrepreneurs are able to work for long periods. Since eight-hour days and 40-hour weeks are simply insufficient to accomplish all that must be done, entrepreneurs must invest more time and more mental and physical energy in the business. They almost never take the time to be sick: they often work in spite of colds and headaches.

In self-descriptions, entrepreneurs generally say that they are high-energy people who do not require a great deal of sleep. Some recent studies suggest that people with this type of personality are drawn to entrepreneurship. The studies also suggest that the entrepreneurs' resiliency is a result of a manic-depressive temperament, and that this hyperperceptive and hyperenergetic state makes them better able to succeed, because it fosters superior conceptual ability (Fieve, 1987, p. 56). (To forestall unnecessary alarm, keep in mind that a manic-depressive temperament is *not* the same as manic-depressive illness.) Barbara J. Chadwick, of BJC & Associates, describes her strengths in terms that are familiar to entrepreneurs.

> I have abundant energy, a positive attitude, drive, organization skills, and salesmanship. These are the strengths I bring to my business, which

provides inservice education services, program design, and evaluation, meeting management, legal consultation, and promotions and marketing to a variety of institutions. My advice to potential nurse entrepreneurs is, stick to it—it's very satisfying. Be patient with progress made. Toot your own horn.

Need for Achievement

Achievement is the goal of the entrepreneur. Entrepreneurs believe that this achievement is obtainable when they apply their own problem-solving strategies, in their own way, and in their own time. They view attempts by others to "help" or direct the accomplishment as unwelcome intrusions that can only ruin the whole project. Donna Oram's desire for the sense of achievement that comes from owning your projects and their outcome led her to start her own health-care marketing and business development enterprise.

I was tired to working for other people and having my ideas used with no credit or compensation. I was vice president for marketing for a home IV therapy company and struggling with owners who wanted to do my job. I wanted free rein. I'm well organized, and I manage projects efficiently. I'm trustworthy, and I can work with people at all levels of the health-care system. I get the job done in the time frame expected. I know this is what the client wants. I have gained control of my projects. In addition, clients view consultants as experts, so my ideas carry more weight than if I were an employee.

Although entrepreneurs share many characteristics, each one is an individual and approaches the role differently. Certain of these differences are related to gender.

GENDER DIFFERENCES

Women do not approach entrepreneurship in precisely the same way that men do, and they often have different reasons for choosing this career path. Although the personality profiles of male and female entrepreneurs are similar, they do not tell the whole story. The realities of a woman's life are vastly different than those of a man's, and these differences give rise to some differences in personal and professional goals and in the methods adopted to achieve these goals through entrepreneurship.

For women, dissatisfaction with work experiences is a prime reason for starting a business. As a group, women business owners are far less likely than men to start a business for the purpose of making a great deal of money or for the thrill of running a giant corporation and wielding great power and influence. They are more concerned with implementing a strategy that will enable them to achieve the flexibility they need to manage the numerous, often conflicting, demands their various roles make on their time and energy. Through entrepreneurship, women seek to achieve success on their own terms: a flexible work role, a wage that enables them to meet their financial obligations, and the freedom to integrate these considerations into their responsibilities to their family. Women tend to view their lives in phases, and business ownership gives them the opportunity to work in sync with these phases (Wojahn, 1986, p. 46). Eva Louise Ransed has discovered the personal satisfactions available in the entrepreneurial role. In 1979, she began her business providing psychotherapy, biofeedback, and consultation to individuals, families, and work systems.

> I was aware that my teaching and clinical positions limited my life and my availability in a way that was unacceptable to me. I saw that other professionals were practicing independently and realized that I had the same abilities. I am able to use my strengths, including my clinical skills, dedication to improve continually, self-discipline, structure, and independence. I have gained the freedom to develop my work as I choose, personal growth, autonomy, and a flexible schedule.

Besides having different reasons for starting a business at all, women entrepreneurs also differ from men entrepreneurs in two respects: (1) management style; and (2) the characteristics of the company built that they build, which include rate of business growth, number of employees, type of business started, amount of outside capital raised, and business location.

Management Style

Most entrepreneurs have only moderate interpersonal skills, and this affects their management style (Welsh & White, 1983, p. 52). Women entrepreneurs, however, traditionally have only been able to exercise power indirectly, and consequently are accustomed to accomplishing goals through the efforts of others. This characteristic enables them to fare better in the growth period, because it makes them good managers. Women business owners are good at rewarding and encouraging employees, problem solving, team building, obtaining input, eliciting information, and achieving consensus. They place great importance on the quality of their relationships with their employees, and thus are more likely than men to consider the needs of individual employees for fulfilling, creative, and satisfying work. Solis (1986) argues that "women bring a broader and more flexible approach [to management] that will be the management theory of the future" (p. 24D). They are concerned about the opinions of others, the respect of their peers, and the satisfaction of their clients. In fact, women managers often play more of a familial role than a managerial one.

The major drawback to this approach is that women business owners often feel that they cannot be successful unless everyone likes them. If carried to an extreme, this feeling may be detrimental. Popular decisions are not always in the best interest of the business.

Characteristics of the Company Built

Women-owned businesses and men-owned businesses grow at different rates. Perhaps because of women's need to balance so many roles and their predisposition to carefully consider the effects of change within the totality of their lives, women-owned business show a slower rate of growth. Integrating such considerations into business decisions suggests that women are more likely to view growth as just one more aspect to juggle in their attempts to achieve a degree of balance in their lives. Since balance is their most important goal, they are likely to view manipulation of the growth rate as a reasonable method of achieving that ultimate goal. For men, the health and growth of the business may be the ultimate goals; for many women, they are not.

The number of people employed by women-run businesses tends to be lower than the number employed by men-run businesses. According to a June 1986 survey of the nation's 500 top small businesses, the average number of full-time employees in a woman's company is 38, whereas the average number in men-run businesses is 130 (Hartman, 1986, p. 54). The reason for this disparity is not known, but it seems likely that if it is present in the largest companies in the country, it is also present in small businesses, too.

Of the many factors that may contribute to the tendency for women business owners to employ fewer workers, three seem especially likely. First, women are twice as likely as men to depend on family finances as a source of operating capital (Hartman, 1986, p. 54). Thus, their decisions about the monetary aspects of the business may tend to be conservative, since these decisions have a direct effect of the financial security of the family.

Second, 40 percent of the businesses that women start are in the service sector ("1986," 1986, p. 35). The profit margin is lower in service-oriented businesses, the competition is greater, and the entry barriers are low, which means that these businesses do not generate capital easily. Women are three times more likely to run their tiny businesses from their home than men are (Wojahn, 1986, p. 46), and, because they do not have their own buildings and a good-sized payroll, they are not in contention for significant amounts of outside capital. Among the largest of the small companies, the *Inc.* 500

companies, the average amount of outside capital raised by women is $91,390, whereas the average amount of outside capital raised by men is $2,177,490 (Hartman, 1986, p. 54).

Third, women tend not to be gamblers. For most women, experience with money has revolved around budgeting, rationing, and conserving it, not using it as a tool for generating additional money.

Consider these gender differences as you analyze your entrepreneurial characteristics, since they may influence your particular style. We are all different even though we are pursuing a common goal, entrepreneurship. For this reason, you must change the broad picture of the entrepreneur we have provided into a self-portrait before you can use the information skillfully.

ENTREPRENEURIAL SELF-ASSESSMENT

As an entrepreneur, you are your own most important asset. Since you are intrinsically linked with your business, your unique personality has a direct impact on its success. Therefore, an assessment of your strengths and limitations and a comparison of your personal characteristics with those usually attributed to successful entrepreneurs are essential to prebusiness planning. In addition, research has demonstrated that entrepreneurial characteristics can be developed. The self-discovery process outlined in this chapter is therefore a crucial step in your personal growth. As you identify your competencies and limitations, you can plan ways of acquiring the personal resources or skills needed for a successful career.

The six assessments below will increase your understanding of your entrepreneurial personality. They cover the following areas:

1. entrepreneurial orientation/internal locus of control,
2. critical event,
3. personal characteristics,
4. interpersonal skills,
5. business and management skills, and
6. nursing expertise.

Following each activity, there is an interpretation of the score and a discussion of methods for acquiring or enhancing essential competencies.

Assessment 2.1 The Entrepreneurial Orientation Inventory

Instructions. This inventory contains 20 pairs of statements. In each pair, you may agree with one statement more than the other. You have five points to distribute between the two statements in each pair, to indicate the extent to which you agree with each of the statements. You may distribute the five points in any combination (0/5, 1/4, 2/3, 4/1, 5/0). If you agree slightly more with statement "a" than with "b," then assign three points to "a" and two points to "b". If you agree very much with "a" and very little with "b," assign four points to "a" and one point to "b". If you agree completely with "a" but do not agree at all with "b," assign five points to "a" and zero to "b". You may not divide your points equally (i.e., 2.5/2.5) between the two choices: You must choose one statement with which you agree more and then distribute the points.

Statement	Points
1.a. How successful an entrepreneur one will be depends on a number of factors. One's capabilities may have very little to do with one's success.	_______
b. A capable entrepreneur can always shape his or her own destiny.	_______
2.a. Entrepreneurs are born, not made.	_______
b. It is possible for people to learn to become more enterprising even if they do not start out that way.	_______
3.a. Whether or not a salesperson will be able to sell his or her product depends on how effective the competitors are.	_______
b. No matter how good the competitors are, an effective salesperson always will be able to sell his or her product.	_______
4.a. Capable entrepreneurs believe in planning their activities in advance.	_______
b. There is no need for advance planning, because no matter how enterprising one is, there always will be chance factors that influence success.	_______

Statement	Points
5.a. Whether or not a person can become a successful entrepreneur depends on social and economic conditions.	______
b. Real entrepreneurs always can be successful, irrespective of social and economic conditions.	______
6.a. Entrepreneurs fail because of their own lack of ability and perspective.	______
b. Entrepreneurs are bound to fail at least half the time, because success or failure depends on a number of factors beyond their control.	______
7.a. Entrepreneurs are often victims of forces that they can neither understand nor control.	______
b. By taking an active part in economic, social, and political affairs, entrepreneurs can control events that affect their businesses.	______
8.a. Whether or not you get a business loan depends on how fair the bank officer you deal with is.	______
b. Whether or not you get a business loan depends on how good your project plan is.	______
9.a. When purchasing raw materials or any other goods, it is wise to collect as much information as possible from various sources and then to make a final choice.	______
b. There is no point in collecting a lot of information; in the long run, the more you pay, the better the product is.	______
10.a. Whether or not you make a profit in business depends on how lucky you are.	______
b. Whether or not you make a profit in business depends on how capable you are as an entrepreneur.	______
11.a. Some types of people can never be successful as entrepreneurs.	______
b. It is possible to develop entrepreneurial ability in different types of people.	______
12.a. Whether or not you will be a successful entrepreneur depends on the social environment into which you were born.	______

Statement	Points
b. People can become successful entrepreneurs with effort and capability, irrespective of the social strata from which they originated.	______
13.a. These days, people must depend at every point on the help, support, or mercy of others (governmental agencies, bureaucracies, banks, etc.).	______
b. It is possible to generate one's own income without depending too much on the bureaucracy. What is required is a knack in dealing with people.	______
14.a. The market situation today is very unpredictable. Even perceptive entrepreneurs falter quite often.	______
b. When an entrepreneur's prediction of the market situation is wrong, that person can blame only himself or herself for failing to read the market correctly.	______
15.a. With effort, people can determine their own destinies.	______
b. There is no point in spending time planning or doing things to change one's destiny. What is going to happen will happen.	______
16.a. There are many events beyond the control of entrepreneurs.	______
b. Entrepreneurs are the creators of their own experiences.	______
17.a. No matter how hard a person works, he or she will achieve only what is destined.	______
b. The rewards one achieves depend solely on the effort one makes.	______
18.a. Organizational effectiveness can be achieved by employing competent and effective people.	______
b. No matter how competent the employees in a company are, if socioeconomic conditions are not good, the organization will have problems.	______
19.a. Leaving things to chance and letting time take care of them helps a person to relax and enjoy life.	______

Statement	Points
b. Working for things always turns out better than leaving things to chance.	______
20.a. The work of competent people always will be recognized.	______
b. No matter how competent one is, it is almost impossible to get ahead in life without contacts.	______

The Entrepreneurial Orientation Inventory Scoring Sheet

Instructions. Transfer your point allocations from the inventory form onto this scoring sheet.

Internal Locus of Control	External Locus of Control
1b	1a
2b	2a
3b	3a
4a	4b
5b	5a
6a	6b
7b	7a
8b	8a
9a	9b
10b	10a
11b	11a
12b	12a

Internal Locus of Control	External Locus of Control
13b	13a
14b	14a
15a	15b
16b	16a
17b	17a
18a	18b
19b	19a
20a	20b
Total internal ______	Total external ______

Determine the ratios of your internal/external locus of control scores by dividing the total internal score by the total external score. Record the amount here ______.

Internal/external ratios above 3.0 indicate a high level of entrepreneurial internality; the chances are high that such individuals will initiate entrepreneurial activities. Ratios below 1.0 indicate that the respondent has a more external (less entrepreneurial) locus-of-control orientation. There is a need for this type of person to become more internal in order to be able to initiate and sustain entrepreneurial activities. Ratios above 1.0 indicate possible entrepreneurs. The higher the ratio above 1.0, the more internal the respondent is.

Reprinted from Rao (1985). Used with permission.

If your score indicates a strong internal locus of control, then you believe in your ability to make things happen. You will persevere in your efforts to reach desired outcomes and take steps to remedy any deficiencies you might have through active acquisition of the necessary knowledge and skills. You tend to be highly motivated to achieve and convinced that you can achieve through your own efforts. Successful entrepreneurs have an internal locus of control.

Persons with an external locus of control tend to attribute the outcome of their actions to chance, luck, their social system, or other factors (Pareek, 1982). They are less likely to persevere, since they do not believe their efforts will affect the outcomes of their actions. Entrepreneurship demands the self-confident pursuit of desirable goals and is a difficult experience for individuals with an external locus of control.

Internalization can be developed, and if your score indicates a tendency towards externalization, there are steps you can take to change your orientation.

1. Self awareness is the first stage in this change process. Monitoring your own behaviors and recognizing patterns that should be modified will provide direction for learning new skills.
2. Use assertiveness training to develop personal strengths, improve self-concept, and gain verbal and nonverbal self-presentation skills.
3. Belonging to a support group or starting individual counseling can enhance your self awareness and restructure the way you interpret internal and external environments.
4. Establish a collaborative relationship or partnership with another entrepreneur who has a strong internal locus of control. Develop a feedback process with this person so that you can continue your own development and eliminate unwanted behaviors.

Assessment 2.2 Critical Event

Instructions. Answer as honestly as you can. Rate yourself from 0 to 6 on each question. A score of 0 means that the statement is never true for you; a score of 6 means that the statement is always true for you. Numerical scores of 1,2,3,4, and 5 represent intermediate scores and are used of statements that are neither all true or all false.

Statement	Score: Never True … Always True
1. I feel that my career is at a standstill.	0 1 2 3 4 5 6
2. It bugs me that I must spend time at work on things I don't think are important.	0 1 2 3 4 5 6

Statement	Score						
	Never True						Always True
3. My chances for advancement in my present job are limited.	0	1	2	3	4	5	6
4. I do not have the option to be creative in my present position.	0	1	2	3	4	5	6
5. I want to make more money.	0	1	2	3	4	5	6
6. I don't feel a sense of achievement in my work.	0	1	2	3	4	5	6
7. My present job isn't fun anymore.	0	1	2	3	4	5	6
8. I'm in a state of personal change now.	0	1	2	3	4	5	6
9. My physical health or a disability has left me "unemployable" in the conventional sense.	0	1	2	3	4	5	6
10. I have been fired, or I may be fired, or I may have to quit my present position.	0	1	2	3	4	5	6
11. I want more independence than I have in my present role.	0	1	2	3	4	5	6
12. I need more control over my work schedule.	0	1	2	3	4	5	6
13. My last birthday was a "traumatic life event" (30, 40, 50+).	0	1	2	3	4	5	6
14. My attempt to balance work and personal roles is creating a high stress level for me.	0	1	2	3	4	5	6

Scoring. Add your scores for the 14 statements. If you scored 65 or more points, you are probably enduring a life or work role that leaves you dissatisfied and unfulfilled. The likelihood of your changing to an entrepreneurial role is high. Any additional negative change in your life or job may provide the catalyst for this transition. If you scored 31 to 64, you may still be interested in a career change, but may be willing to wait before making a move. If you scored 0 to 30, your present life and work roles provide satisfaction. You may still want to be an entrepreneur, but you do not feel strongly compelled to do it now.

For many individuals, the option of starting a business on a small scale while maintaining a job that offers moderate rewards is a realistic option. Consider this possibility if you are prevented from making a total change for personal or financial reasons.

Assessment 2.3 Personal Characteristics

Instructions. Answer as honestly as you can. Rate yourself on each statement using a scale of 0 to 6. A score of 0 means that the statement is never true for you; a score of 6 means that it is always true. For each of the following 34 statements, place a check under the column that represents your numerical score for that statement. A score of 6 indicates exceptional capacity; a score of 4 or 5 indicates well-developed competencies; a score of 2 or 3 indicates undeveloped areas that may interfere with your ability to function in an entrepreneurial role; and a score of 0 or 1 represents a deficiency of greater magnitude that may adversely affect your performance as an entrepreneur.

	Rating			
Statement	Deficient (0,1)	Under-developed (2,3)	Well-Developed (4,5)	Exceptional (6)
1. Even when I was young, I had business ventures.				
2. As a youngster, I had entrepreneurial role models—parents, neighbors.				
3. I have friends and contacts who are entrepreneurs.				

Statement	Rating: Deficient (0,1)	Under-developed (2,3)	Well-Developed (4,5)	Exceptional (6)
4. I can visualize myself in an independent, entrepreneurial role.				
5. I'm willing to take risks that I view as reasonable.				
6. I enjoy ambiguity because it stimulates my creativity.				
7. I have more energy than most people I know.				
8. I'm a critical thinker.				
9. I have a good sense of humor and can laugh at myself.				
10. The respect and admiration of others is important to me, but it does not deter me from taking an unpopular stand or pursuing goals that are important to me.				

	Rating			
Statement	Deficient (0,1)	Under-developed (2,3)	Well-Developed (4,5)	Exceptional (6)
11. I'm usually the one in my work group who initiates new ways of solving old problems.				
12. I like the challenge of new tasks or projects.				
13. I prefer to have the sole accountability for project outcomes.				
14. I will work extremely hard at problems or tasks when I believe I can make a difference in how they turn out.				
15. I'm good at influencing others to accept new ways of doing things.				
16. I'm comfortable marketing myself or my ideas to others.				
17. I'm good at "networking."				

Statement	Rating: Deficient (0,1)	Under-developed (2,3)	Well-Developed (4,5)	Exceptional (6)
18. I don't worry about the limits of my job description, but take the initiative to implement my role.				
19. I like to consider possibilities rather than limitations.				
20. I frequently see the problems inherent in a system and look for ways to overcome them or change the system.				
21. Other people ask for my help or advice in matters related to my special skills.				
22. I reward myself when I feel I've done a good job.				
23. I've found ways to take care of my needs for positive feedback.				

Statement	Rating: Deficient (0,1)	Under-developed (2,3)	Well-Developed (4,5)	Exceptional (6)
24. The biggest reward I have from my work is self-actualization.				
25. I prefer independence in my work role.				
26. I prefer variety in my work.				
27. I can mobilize necessary resources (time, people, energy) when a job needs to get done.				
28. I enjoy responsibility.				
29. Although I prefer autonomy, I can collaborate well with others on work projects.				
30. I can usually find new opportunities to use my skills.				
31. I learn from my failures.				
32. I know how to relax when my stress level gets too high.				

Statement	Rating: Deficient (0,1)	Under-developed (2,3)	Well-Developed (4,5)	Exceptional (6)
33. I'm discreet and do not share information inappropriately.				
34. I can deal with loneliness.				

Statements 4, 5, 9, 14, 16, 22, 23, 31, 32, and 34 assess self-concept; statements 15, 17, 21, 27, 29, and 33 assess leadership influence; statements 7, 10, 13, 18, 24, 25, and 28 assess independence, drive, and desire; and statements 6, 8, 11, 12, 19, 20, 26, and 30 assess creativity and problem solving.

The first three statements represent personal experiences with entrepreneurs or entrepreneurship that give you special insights into the role. If you lack these experiences, you may be well advised to work with a partner, seek out a mentor, or develop an entrepreneurial network for support and feedback. The fourth statement indicates how much you believe in yourself as an entrepreneur. The remaining 30 items address the skills and traits listed above.

Scoring. If most of your checks are in the "well-developed" or "exceptional" categories, you have the drive, creativity, insights, and personal strengths to handle the entrepreneurial role. Deficiencies or underdeveloped traits require reflection on your part. Carefully consider the effect that lack of any given characteristic may have on your capacity to function as an entrepreneur. If the deficiencies are likely to be problematic, steps should be formulated and implemented to diminish their capacity to hinder your performance.

Skills can be developed in several ways. Workshops, credit courses, and independent reading are three useful strategies. Collaboration with someone who has the skills you lack is also helpful. Consultation with a peer group or a mentor as you begin your new career can provide the support and feedback you need to grow.

Assessment 2.4 Interpersonal Skills

Entrepreneurs experience a special dilemma: whereas they crave independence, they also understand the need for collaborative problem solving if their own and their clients' goals are to be attained effectively. Because collaboration is so important, successful entrepreneurs must rely heavily on their interpersonal skills. In this assessment, you will determine the extent to which you possess these skills.

Instructions. Using the same 0 to 6 scale described in Assessment 2.2, rate yourself on each of the following 15 statements.

Statement	Score Never True … Always True
1. I tune in to other people's verbal and nonverbal messages when I'm listening to them.	0 1 2 3 4 5 6
2. I have excellent verbal and nonverbal self-presentation skills.	0 1 2 3 4 5 6
3. I can express abstract concepts in concrete terms.	0 1 2 3 4 5 6
4. I clarify and validate messages when communicating with others.	0 1 2 3 4 5 6
5. I am comfortable confronting another person in a conflict situation.	0 1 2 3 4 5 6
6. I can set limits on how other people use my time.	0 1 2 3 4 5 6
7. I can say no.	0 1 2 3 4 5 6
8. I can tell others about my limitations as well as my strengths.	0 1 2 3 4 5 6
9. I can establish problem ownership when resolving conflicts with others.	0 1 2 3 4 5 6
10. I'm an effective group facilitator.	0 1 2 3 4 5 6
11. People frequently seek me out for help with interpersonal or work problems.	0 1 2 3 4 5 6
12. I use power skillfully.	0 1 2 3 4 5 6

Statement	Score Never True … Always True
13. I can effectively handle other people's attempts to use their power inappropriately with me.	0 1 2 3 4 5 6
14. Even in a conflict situation, I use an assertive style that preserves others' integrity as well as my own.	0 1 2 3 4 5 6
15. I'm a good negotiator.	0 1 2 3 4 5 6

Scoring. Which skills do you need to develop? The numerical scores for each statement can be interpreted in much the same way as in Assessment 2.3 (i.e., deficient, underdeveloped, well-developed, or exceptional).

Assessment 2.5 Business and Management Skills

As an entrepreneur, you know that owning and managing your own business requires special expertise. This assessment enables you to evaluate your strengths in this area.

Instructions. Using the 0 to 6 scale employed in Assessments 2.2, 2.3, and 2.4, rate yourself on each of the following 15 statements.

Statement	Score Never True … Always True
1. I see the "big picture" even when I'm working on a small part of the total problem.	0 1 2 3 4 5 6
2. I regularly establish goals and timetables.	0 1 2 3 4 5 6
3. I consistently look for patterns or trends in the external environment so that I can plan changes.	0 1 2 3 4 5 6

Statement	Score Never True … Always True
4. I regularly check where I am in the process of meeting target dates for my goals.	0 1 2 3 4 5 6
5. I can be flexible and switch my goals when new demands or priorities occur.	0 1 2 3 4 5 6
6. I regularly set aside planning time.	0 1 2 3 4 5 6
7. I plan daily how I can best use my time to meet my goals.	0 1 2 3 4 5 6
8. I'm an organized person.	0 1 2 3 4 5 6
9. I can coordinate several complex activities and keep everything running smoothly.	0 1 2 3 4 5 6
10. I can put a price on what I provide and ask for reimbursement for my service.	0 1 2 3 4 5 6
11. I can list my financial assets and liabilities.	0 1 2 3 4 5 6
12. I know where to find capital for a new venture.	0 1 2 3 4 5 6
13. I have fund-raising experience.	0 1 2 3 4 5 6
14. I have good accounting skills.	0 1 2 3 4 5 6
15. I understand marketing concepts.	0 1 2 3 4 5 6

Your business and management skills can be developed by means of the techniques listed in the previous assessments. As alternatives, three other strategies may be tried.

1. Use a professional expert, such as a lawyer, accountant, or marketing analyst, to get expert advice.
2. If you are not ready to leave your present job just yet, seek out new experiences in your current role that will allow you to learn and practice business and management skills.
3. Volunteer for activities (community efforts, work, professional associations, or hobbies) that will permit you to develop specialized competencies.

Assessment 2.6 Nursing Expertise

As a nurse entrepreneur, you are marketing something very special: your professional nursing expertise. Your clients will expect you to understand the intrinsic nature of nursing and its unique role in today's health-care systems. In this assessment, you will evaluate the degree to which you maintain the ideals of professionalism in your nursing practice.

Instructions. Rate yourself on each of the following 15 statements using the 0 to 6 scale implemented in the previous four assessments.

Statement	Score: Never True ... Always True
1. I maintain a consistent pattern of continuing education.	0 1 2 3 4 5 6
2. I can explain how I integrate nursing theory as a framework for my practice with clients.	0 1 2 3 4 5 6
3. I conduct or utilize the results of research as a basis for change in the way I implement my role.	0 1 2 3 4 5 6
4. I establish client relationships by mutually defining goals for care or interventions.	0 1 2 3 4 5 6
5. I utilize nursing diagnosis as a basis for care with patients.	0 1 2 3 4 5 6
6. I belong to a professional organization.	0 1 2 3 4 5 6
7. I am active in a professional organization.	0 1 2 3 4 5 6
8. I act as an advocate for the role of professional nursing.	0 1 2 3 4 5 6
9. I act as a patient advocate.	0 1 2 3 4 5 6
10. I can establish effective client relationships.	0 1 2 3 4 5 6
11. I keep current with what happens in professional nursing.	0 1 2 3 4 5 6

Statement	Score Never True … Always True
12. I have had successful leadership positions in nursing.	0 1 2 3 4 5 6
13. I have a broad base of professional contacts in the community.	0 1 2 3 4 5 6
14. I am experienced in helping others learn.	0 1 2 3 4 5 6
15. I actively implement a quality assurance process as part of my professional role.	0 1 2 3 4 5 6

Scoring. Add your scores for the 15 statements. A total score of 75 to 90 indicates that your credibility and marketability as a nurse expert are excellent. A score of 45 to 74 indicates that you might experience difficulty in being recognized as a nurse expert by potential clients. A score of less than 45 indicates that nursing clients are relatively unlikely to identify you as a nurse expert. Since your credibility as a nurse expert has a direct impact on your ability to influence others, low scores here should encourage you to expand your knowledge. Each of the statements suggests a strategy for broadening your nursing expertise.

The self-knowledge gained through this series of assessments is in itself a source of strength. Enumerating your skills enhances your self-concept, and understanding your limitations equips you to plan to eliminate them or reduce their impact. The end result of your hard work in this chapter is a strategic plan for developing your unique entrepreneurial personality. Before proceeding to chapter 3, complete Exercise 2.1.

✔ Exercise 2.1 Entrepreneurial Personality Profile.

Instructions. Use the self-knowledge acquired in Assessments 2.1 through 2.6 to complete this exercise. Review your assessment answers, and fill out both part I and part II.

Part I is concerned with your strengths. Identify your personality strengths and explain how they will enhance your ability to function as an entrepreneur.

My Strengths	How They Will Increase My Ability to Function

Part II is concerned with your limitations. List the limitations you have, and indicate how you plan to eliminate them or minimize their impact.

My Limitations	Strategies to Eliminate or Reduce Impact

With an awareness of your strengths and limitations, you can initiate the journey toward independence by acquiring essential skills and finding mentors in other nurse entrepreneurs. As your entrepreneurial orientation expands, your desire to find a niche for yourself in this new career environment is strengthened. The next chapter will help you locate new opportunities and find that niche.

3 FINDING A NICHE

Once you choose an entrepreneurial option, how do you find your niche? In other words, how do you transform a business idea into a marketable outlet for your unique talents? There are several strategies for finding the right niche, but the most important one is, *provide the right service to the right market.*

Although this strategy may sound simple enough, implementing it requires continual assessment of current and emerging problems in your clients' milieu and the establishment of a relationship between those problems and your business ideas. A client-centered approach is imperative, because your business survival depends on your ability to meet client-dictated rather than provider-dictated needs. From the day you get your first client, you must find out why he or she is your client. Why does the client buy your service/product? What does the client find appealing about it? Why has the client chosen you instead of the competition? Does the client have any suggestions as to how your service/product could be made even more appealing? Knowing your customers well helps you to tailor your marketing efforts to specific target groups, research target groups' present and future needs, estimate the potential size of your current market, and project the growth of that market over the next five years. Your clients' needs may be unmet or poorly met, clearly articulated or vaguely implied. If you are to be a successful entrepreneur, however, you must be able to interpret them accurately, match them with your special skills, and market services that specifically address them.

Finding the right niche involves a series of steps, each one a preparation for the next: (1) developing a business idea, (2) performing a market-service analysis, (3) market testing, and (4) launching a trial balloon. For some nurses, like Donna Ipema, of Associates in Counseling, this process is rapid and fairly simple.

> I recognized that as I moved from one agency to another (for geographical proximity), my psychotherapy clients followed me. I also realized that client referral was building my practice. My training as a psychiatric nurse makes me a unique provider, since I understand the interaction

> between physical and psychological problems. For these reasons, I knew the market was there and didn't do any market testing when I started my practice in 1981.

For many nurse entrepreneurs, however, the process of finding their niche will have to be considerably more complex and deliberative. The four steps listed above, if carefully followed as described below, should alleviate that complexity to some extent.

DEVELOPING A BUSINESS IDEA

A business idea is a seed from which a successful enterprise grows. That growth cannot occur, however, until the initial idea is refined into a business statement that describes services or products, potential clients, and realistic business goals.

Refining a Business Idea

Your idea may be nothing more complicated than "I want to have my own business." You may have ideas about a variety of services or products that you could offer as an entrepreneur, or you may have a single idea that is so good it is bound to work. Whatever your situation, you must transform the initial concept into a business statement.

If you are starting with a desire to be an entrepreneur but are unsure what services you want to offer, ask yourself what you most enjoy doing or what you are most skilled at doing. Through close self-examination, try to determine

- what skills you have,
- what skills you enjoy using,
- what skills or activities you dislike,
- what environment you prefer to work in, and
- what lifestyle and income you require.

One approach to identifying your skills is to write a story about an event in your life that relates to something you accomplished or a situation in which you particularly enjoyed yourself. Next, review the story, and identify the skills that are obvious or can be inferred from the verbs you used. These skills may involve working with people, information, or things. Figures 3.1, 3.2, and 3.3 contain numerous possible transferrable skills in each of these domains, listed in a hierarchy with the most complex skills at the top. Review these figures to determine what skills you most want to use as an entrepreneur.

Another approach to identifying your skills is to write a summary of your background experience. This approach can help you to pinpoint skill deficits, as well as encourage you to think about the kinds of skills you would like to use in your entrepreneurial role.

Hobbies, avocations, and social and educational involvements are other sources of ideas about the skills you have and like to use. It is often possible to build many of these activities into your new role. Awareness of your dislikes is equally important, since your ideal job can be structured to avoid many aspects of work you find tedious or onerous.

The environment in which you would like to work includes the geographic region; the type of business—manufacturing, retail, or service, indoors or outdoors; the level of responsibility expected; the extent of autonomy allowed; and the degree of structure present. All these aspects must be considered and prioritized if you are to make a fully informed decision.

The lifestyle and income you want also affect how you structure your role. List the things that are important to you: Do you want a home in the

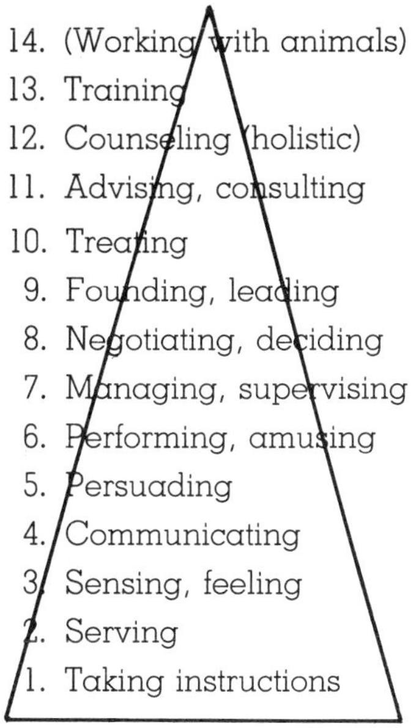

14. (Working with animals)
13. Training
12. Counseling (holistic)
11. Advising, consulting
10. Treating
9. Founding, leading
8. Negotiating, deciding
7. Managing, supervising
6. Performing, amusing
5. Persuading
4. Communicating
3. Sensing, feeling
2. Serving
1. Taking instructions

Figure 3.1 Skills that primarily involve people, though they may also involve information and things. (From Bolles, 1986, p. 230. Used with permission.)

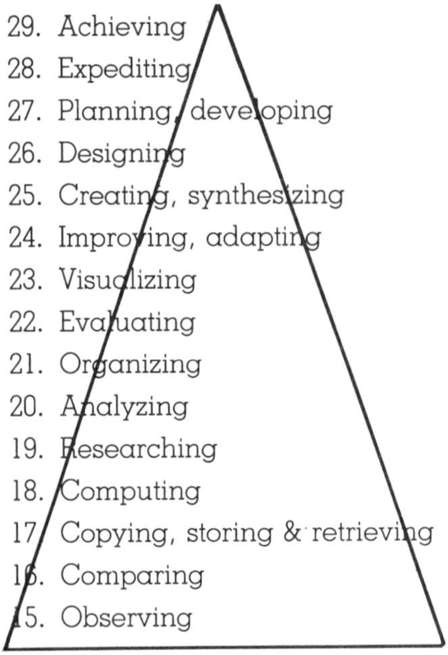

29. Achieving
28. Expediting
27. Planning, developing
26. Designing
25. Creating, synthesizing
24. Improving, adapting
23. Visualizing
22. Evaluating
21. Organizing
20. Analyzing
19. Researching
18. Computing
17. Copying, storing & retrieving
16. Comparing
15. Observing

Figure 3.2 Skills that primarily involve information or data, though they may also involve things. (From Bolles, 1986, p. 230. Used with permission.)

40. Repairing
39. Setting up
38. Precision working
37. Operating (vehicles)
36. Operating (equipment)
35. Using (tools)
34. Minding (machines)
33. Feeding, emptying (machines)
32. Working with the earth or nature
31. Being athletic
30. Handling (objects)

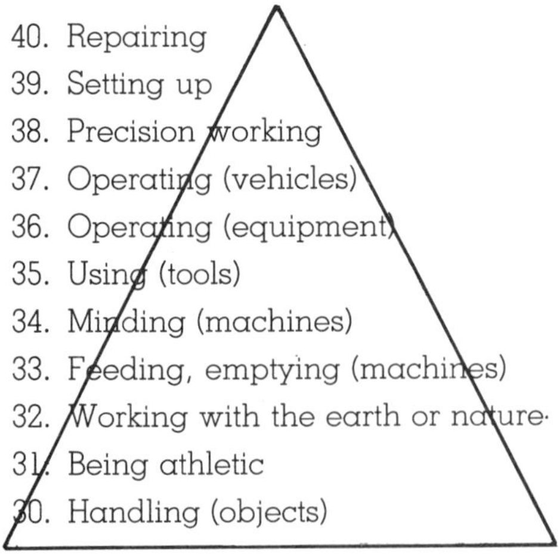

Figure 3.3 Skills that primarily involve things, though they may also involve information. (From Bolles, 1986, p. 230. Used with permission.)

south of France? three Mercedes-Benzes? private schools for your children? a business you can run part-time for two years? a business you can expand into a chain across the country? a business you can franchise? a business where you can use your talents and experiences without a boss? Prioritize all your preferences, so that the most important aspects are not lost as the role is structured. Incorporate these criteria into your initial business goals.

✔ Exercise 3.1 Choice of Skills.

This is the appropriate time to decide which skills you want to use in your new role and which skills or activities you want to avoid.

Instructions. List the requested information under each of the columns below.

1. In my role as an entrepreneur I want to be able to use the following skills or engage in the following activities.

Skills	Activities

2. In my role as an entrepreneur, I want to avoid having to do the following tasks or activities.

Tasks	Activities

Keep these lists in mind as you proceed with this chapter and search for your entrepreneurial niche.

If you have some idea what you would like to do, it may be helpful to study what is required of people who are successfully engaged in that activity. If you think you might like consulting, for example, Exercise 3.2 should give you additional insight into this career.

Exercise 3.2 The Consultant's Role.

The following 38 phrases represent salient aspects of the consultant's business role that are frequently encountered.

Instructions. Rate how satisfying these role aspects are in the work you do. 1 = satisfying, 0 = neutral, −1 = unsatisfying.

Role Aspect	Score
1. Creating or contributing new ideas	______
2. Communication in many forms (verbal, written) with various people	______
3. Advising rather than directing others	______
4. Taking initiative to both start and complete tasks	______
5. Working in new and different locations on a regular basis	______
6. Utilizing positive interpersonal skills to accomplish tasks	______
7. Having little job security	______
8. Inspiring confidence in your judgments	______
9. Not doing the same things all the time	______
10. Managing people, projects, and paperwork on a regular basis	______
11. Being respected by others	______
12. Finding yourself in ambiguous, undefined relationships	______
13. Meeting new people and new situations	______
14. Possessing an expertise in a specific area	______
15. Opportunity for high economic return	______
16. Listening continually and sincerely to others' verbal and nonverbal messages	______
17. Working best without supervision	______

Role Aspect	Score
18. Having credibility as a result of expertise, experience, or credentials	______
19. Having to keep solving new problems	______
20. Learning new ideas and applying them	______
21. Constant travel, resulting in prolonged periods away from home	______
22. Feeling you have helped other people	______
23. Holding strong ethical values concerning the conduct of your work	______
24. Seeing your ideas rejected or not implemented	______
25. Working alone for the most part	______
26. Selling your services to others	______
27. Working long and hard hours until project is completed	______
28. Engaging in self-reflection in order to learn from experience	______
29. Being responsible for the quality and usefulness of your work	______
30. Understanding and utilizing organizational dynamics	______
31. Understanding the motivation behind other people's behavior	______
32. Maintaining objectivity in planning and carrying out assignments	______
33. Maintaining confidentiality about your client's business problems	______
34. Being well organized in approaching and completing assignments	______
35. Having better than average ability to recognize, describe, and solve problems	______
36. Being a high-energy, ambitious person	______
37. Working effectively on several projects simultaneously	______
38. Being creative and confident in approaching problems that seem to have no resolution	______

Scoring. Add up all the scores. A total score of 20 to 38 indicates that you meet the major requirements of consulting. A score of 0 to 19 indicates a moderate suitability to consulting. A score of −1 to −38 indicates poor suitability to consulting. (Phrases 1 to 30 are taken from Kelley, 1981, pp. 12–14.)

The direct approach to people you would like to emulate is highly effective. Frequently we hesitate to telephone them, make an appointment with them, or take them out to lunch because we fear our overtures will be rejected. At times, you will indeed get a resounding "No!" to your request for information, or the person you contact will hang up on you. Far more often, however, successful entrepreneurs are glad to share information with you. They are generally willing to tell you about their business, and they may well offer valuable suggestions for your potential business venture. The letter reproduced in Figure 3.4 was written recently in response to a stranger's request for information about Advanced Health Care Concepts and for advice on her business idea.

Trying to work through several business ideas at once creates as many problems as an idea deficit does. Suzanne Hall Johnson, director of Hall Johnson Communications, Inc., is an experienced nurse entrepreneur who advises new entrepreneurs to avoid the multiple service trap.

> A common mistake that new entrepreneurs make is offering too many different services at once. Their energy is dispersed, and they become exhausted. Develop one service at a time, and do not add a new service until the first one is going well with little attention.

If you have several business ideas, the content and exercises in the remainder of this chapter will help you select the one idea that represents the most viable business opportunity. Even when you are certain that yours is the "winning idea," it is essential to evaluate that idea's potential marketability before you make a major investment of financial and energy resources.

A winning idea must be unique in some way, whether because it is totally new, because it is an improvement on an existing concept, because it is a better method for delivery or financing, or because it is a duplication of an existing business in a new area. Laura Gasparis, of CPR Associates, has a unique delivery factor that increases the marketability of her business.

> I provide CPR education to large companies (i.e., E.F. Hutton), small companies, doctors, attorneys, walk-in clinics, schools, catering halls, etc. Our product is not unique; our availability is. We train at the participant's place of employment as well as market "CPR parties." During our market testing, letters were sent to two large corporations, and we received a positive response—requests to train 1,000 people in CPR.

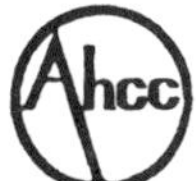

ADVANCED HEALTH CARE CONCEPTS

3799 TURNWOOD DRIVE, RICHFIELD, WISCONSIN 53076

October 14, 1986

Ms. xxxxxxxxxxxx, R.N., M.S.
Clinical Nurse Specialist
xxxxxxxxxxxx
xxxxxxxxxxxx
xxxxxxxxxxxx, Tennessee xxxxx

Dear Ms. xxxxx:

In response to your letter of 9/25/86, I am happy to share with you information about Advanced Health Care Concepts and to make a few recommendations regarding your venture.

Advanced Health Care Concepts (AHCC) started in June 1980 as a partnership. The purpose of the venture was to provide nursing experts on an ''as needed'' basis wherever such expertise is needed, e.g., institutions, corporations, and service corporations. The premise underlying the creation of this company was that nursing expertise and patient care in southeastern Wisconsin (my little corner of the world) would be improved via this access. Every institution could have as much of any particular expertise as they required when they needed it. I thought this to be important, because most patient care institutions cannot afford to hire as many nursing specialists as they need. Many do without any clinical nurse specialists, or they end up trying to hire a medical-surgical CNS and then make him or her responsible for the quality of all nursing care throughout the entire institution! (For further insights into AHCC, I have included a copy of my article entitled ''The Role of the Nurse Consultant in Enhancing Practice Skills'' and a column ''Meet an Alum,'' which is due to be published in my school of nursing alumni newsletter 4/87.)

Until 8/81, I continued to work part-time as a clinical nurse specialist in neuro/ortho/trauma. After that date, AHCC became my full-time career. The partnership was dissolved at that time, and the business became a proprietorship. There are about 30 clinical nurse specialists who provide services for the company. I subcontract with them, so they are not my employees, and I do not need to be involved with issues such as unemployment compensation, health insurance, worker's compensation, FICA, and other taxes.

The nurses with whom I subcontract continue to work at other jobs elsewhere and maintain their clinical expertise in that way. My own clinical expertise is maintained by staffing in a college of nursing wellness clinic and by functioning as a trauma spe-

Figure 3.4 Sample letter sent in response to a request for information and advice on a business idea.

cialist with the fire department. The role involves being a fully trained fire department member and being on call to participate in search, rescue, extrication, transportation, triage, resuscitation, and the prehospital provision of emergency care. (I don't put out fires.) This commitment is above the 50 or so hours a week I devote to the business.

The specialists usually do consulting or continuing education within their specialty. By way of example, one psychiatric clinical nurse specialist worked with an emergency room staff to help them deal with agitated, confused, combative psychiatric admissions. She helped them develop the skills necessary to avoid confrontation and violence where possible, helped them develop systems for obtaining assistance quickly when such problems were unavoidable, and helped them develop policies and procedures that legitimized their course of action in given situations.

Often times legal mandates are a source of business. When Wisconsin changed its nurse practice act, it mandated nursing diagnosis. This provided numerous jobs preparing nurses to assume this new responsibility and assisting them to develop nursing systems to support the new behavior within their institutions.

The company also presents continuing education programs to the nursing community at large. If you buy the RN list from your state board of nursing, you'll know the name, address, and age of every nurse in the state! You can get this list according to zipcode, which is handy for targeting specific areas. Membership lists from various nursing organizations can be purchased; this helps you zero in on nurses who have special interests. AHCC invested in a computer system which permits lists to be created according to specific variables, such as zipcode or nursing speciality. The computer system also permits literature searches through the National Library of Medicine in Washington, DC, to be done via the telephone and modem in our offices. (A brochure from one of AHCC's early CE programs for the community at large is enclosed.)

Prior to starting the business, a business plan was written. It was very sketchy, but now, after several years in business, it is fully fleshed out—complete with pro forma financial statements! I like a book by Welsh and White called *The Entrepreneur's Master Planning Guide*. It gives examples of what a business plan should have and assistance in putting your plan together. There are more self-helps available now than when this company was started. The public library may have numerous books you need; they may have a small business library.

The Small Business Administration (SBA) in your town undoubtedly offers classes on how to go into business for yourself ($20.00 for six weeks). The SBA also has a group called SCORE—Service Corps Of Retired Executives—to assist (free) with real-life problems new or established business run into. The university extension system probably has a service to help people starting businesses (usually free). There may be a Venture Management Of-

Figure 3.4 continued

fice at your University also. They look at your plan for a nominal fee—$75.00 or so—and tell you what they think your chances are, offering recommendations to make the plan more feasible when needed.

There are some books that deal with nurse-entrepreneurs—have your librarian run a literature search through the National Library of Medicine on the CATLINE. I am coauthoring a book on consulting and entrepreneuring for nurses that is slated for publication in 1987; it is likely that resources will continue to become more available.

You may not be aware of this, but Milwaukee (and Wisconsin) are very conservative areas. When corporations want to know if they can sell a new product, they test market it in Milwaukee. If it flies here, it'll fly anywhere! My company has grown, and I would never give up what I'm doing. I believe that the trends in health care are such that this business can only get bigger and better—even in Wisconsin!

If you haven't read Naisbitt's *Megatrends* and Toffler's *The Third Wave*, I suggest that you do that. Also, get a subscription to the *Wall Street Journal*. Enclosed is an article from Monday's *Wall Street Journal* that has implications for pediatric services. Watch the trends in Colorado and California, since these are bellwether states. Consider whether you want to be intrapreneurs or entrepreneurs—this will make all the difference in how you set up the business. Consider marketing your services directly to health care consumers (mothers) and other systems which deal with children. You might, for example, make videotapes on promoting self-esteem in children to assist in stemming the tide of teenage pregnancies and drug abuse in schools.

Investigate the current state of third-party reimbursement for nurses in Tennessee and restrictions regarding service corporations formed by nurses. Also, with the new federal tax law changes coming up, look at subchapter S on incorporations versus C incorporation. You may, by the way, find an existing small business to purchase at a good price because of the unfavorable capital gains taxes that will go into effect on January 1, 1987.

I hope this information is helpful to you. Don't be afraid to call (414-628-0251) or write if I can help you additionally. Good luck in your venture.

Sincerely yours,

Nancy Doleysh, RN, MSN
President, Advanced Health Care Concepts

ND/tom

Enclosures

Figure 3.4 continued

Identifying the unique component of your idea will help you define your competitive edge when you begin market testing that idea.

When properly refined, each business idea becomes a comprehensive statement that describes the service or product, explains what makes it unique, and lists the potential client subgroups (thus making possible accurate definition of target markets). Connie Roethel's description of the business she co-owns is an example of a comprehensive business statement.

> Diabetic Shoppe provides a complete line of diabetic supplies, equipment, medications, skin and foot care products, and foods; nutritional and other educational publications; instruction; and follow-up on all products. Our clients are type I and type II diabetics.

This selection of two subgroups (type I and type II diabetics) from a larger client group (diabetics) clearly delineates the target market. The business statement itself forms the basis for goal setting, which is a marketing prerequisite.

Goal Setting

In our own experience, establishing realistic business goals was as important as fiscal planning, because it provided

- a focus for marketing,
- direction for expenditure of financial and energy resources,
- a yardstick for measuring success and growth, and
- stimulus for change and development of new goals.

The goals that Gerry Vogel developed for WORKSTYLES influenced the product line, the locale, and the pace of business growth over the first two years.

> When I began my business venture, I had several family obligations that were high-priority in terms of where I wanted to spend my time. In addition, I was not known as a management consultant and needed to build credibility for my expertise. I wanted to limit my initial growth during the first two years while preparing to expand when my parenting role ended. Therefore, my initial business goals were to
>
> - develop and present educational programs for nurse managers that would serve as a marketing strategy for future consulting roles,

> - limit business marketing to the state of Wisconsin for the first year to maximize time and energy,
> - contact potential clients within the first three months to increase their awareness of my availability and understanding of the services I offer,
> - publish at least two articles on management-related topics within the first two years to increase my name recognition,
> - develop a brochure within the first 18 months that highlights the consulting aspects of my business,
> - establish a management consulting practice within three years that would allow me to use my team-building and people-development skills to help nurse managers and nursing staff function cohesively and competently.
>
> These goals worked well for me. Within two years, my business expanded at the desired rate, and I was comfortable with the balance I had achieved between my personal and professional roles.

As Nancy Doleysh refined her ideas for Advanced Health Care Concepts, goals evolved that reflected her desire to have an impact on the quality of nursing care and ensure a steady business growth.

> I saw my business as the opportunity to provide expertise to nurses caring for patients. My goals were to
>
> - develop a service which will improve the quality of nursing care by providing affordable access to the expertise of clinical nurse specialists for consultation, education, practice, and research-related activities;
> - develop a holistic approach for all institutional consulting and education-related activities, basing all solutions on an assessment that analyzes needs, institutional culture, and norms and ensures an understanding of the client's goals and desired outcomes;
> - provide an opportunity for individual nurse practitioners to increase their proficiency by presenting workshops with a clinical specialty focus;
> - utilize those clinical experts and educational resources in programming and consulting that will have the greatest impact on clinical practice;
> - develop and offer new product lines as initial services are established; and
> - write a formal business plan to use in the search for venture capital for future business expansion.

Goals keep you on the right path as you work at finding a niche. They should be reevaluated frequently and changed when appropriate. At this stage, they are an integral part of the business definition you will use to complete a market-service analysis. Before proceeding to the next section, use Exercise 3.3 to develop your business idea. If you have several business ideas, complete the exercise for each idea.

✔ Exercise 3.3 Developing A Business Idea.

Instructions. Complete each section in sequence.

1. *Business idea.* What is your business? Describe your business idea as succinctly as possible. What services or products will you offer? What is the unique component of your idea?

2. *Clients.* Who are your clients? List the clients who will use your services. Distinguish between those who will use a service and those who will pay for the service, if the two are different. This distinction has an impact on who makes up your real target market.

Who will use your services?	Who will pay for the services?

3. *Client subgroups.* It is necessary to target client populations as specifically as possible in order to perform a market analysis. Separate your client groups into commonly occurring subgroups. For example, the group "Nurses" could be divided into subgroups on the basis of specialty or role.

   Client group 1:
   Subgroups:

Client group 2:
Subgroups:

Client group 3:
Subgroups:

Client group 4:
Subgroups:

4. *Business Scope*

   a. How extensive a client market do you want? (Give numbers and location.)

      First year:

      Second to fifth year:

   b. How much business do you want to generate?

      First year:

      Second to fifth year:

5. Is your business service/product-driven or client-driven? What methods are you going to implement to ensure that your business is client centered?

6. *Goals.* What are your business goals? These goals can relate to clients, marketing, desired growth, desired income, personal requirements, etc.

You will refine this business idea as you proceed through this chapter.

Goals are the basis for a market-service analysis. As you complete the analysis and develop new insights into potential business opportunities, reexamine your goals, and rewrite them if necessary. The purpose of these exercises is to stimulate creative thinking and generate a richness of options, thereby increasing your chances of finding the right niche.

MARKET-SERVICE ANALYSIS

The market-service analysis model is a tool designed to help you identify client problems and select those services that are most likely to resolve them. A problem exists when there is a gap between what is expected to occur and what is actually occurring. Needs arise from these problems, and your expertise can help meet these needs, resolve the problems, and close the gap.

The model in Figure 3.5 depicts the four components of a market-service analysis: (1) data collection, (2) problem identification, (3) needs analysis selection, and (4) client-centered business focus. Completing such an analysis allows you to transform your business idea into a marketable entity.

Data Collection

The goal of data collection is to generate as many clues as possible about current and emerging client problems. During this stage, you strategically expand information networks while keeping tight focus on the type of information you will need. You can sharpen your focus by continually asking yourself, "What are the problems or needs suggested by this information?" Nurses have three data sources readily available to them: professional experience, personal networks, and literature surveys.

Experience. As an expert professional, you have an insider's view of the impact of changing health-care dynamics on people and systems. Conse-

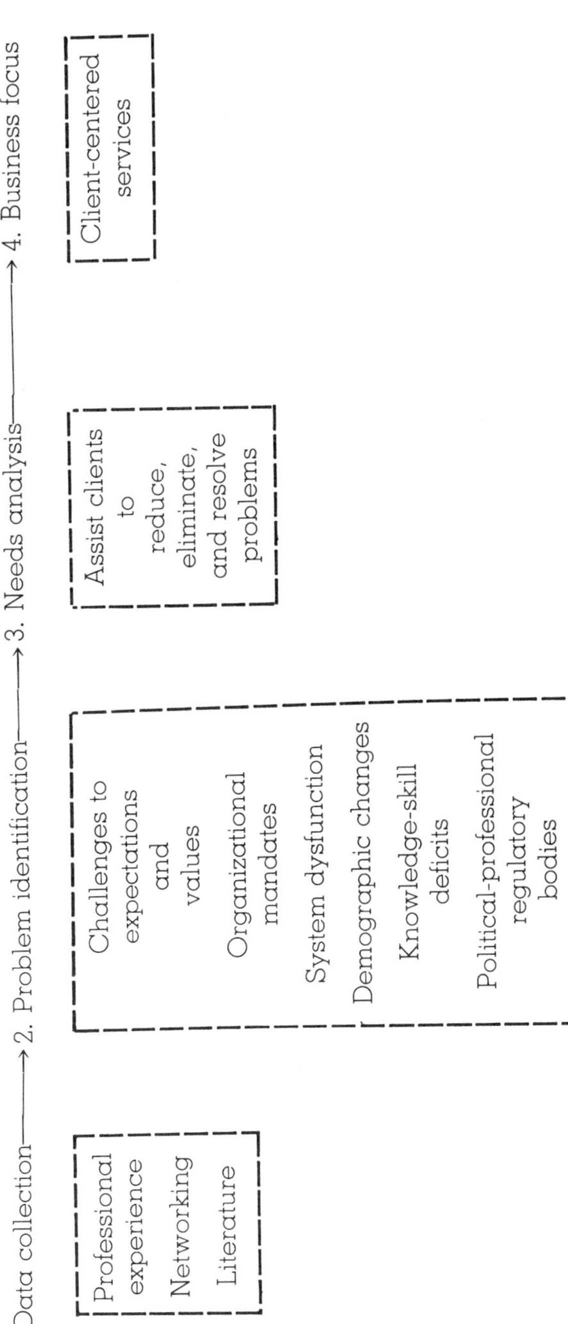

Figure 3.5 A diagram of the market-service analysis process.

quently, your work experience is the source of many business ideas. To capitalize on this opportunity, ask yourself the following questions.

- How is the nursing profession changing, and what impact do these changes have on the needs of others?
- What frustrations do I feel at work?
- What requests for help, information, or advice do I frequently receive from others?
- What problems do I routinely resolve for others?
- What functions of my role could I isolate and market to others?

The answer to such questions can often be transformed into marketable services. Susan R. Donaldson, of Independent Nursing Services, picked up on the cues these answers supply and developed a new business providing private duty nursing services in homes, hospitals, and extended care facilities, as well as staffing in area institutions.

> My original partner, Doris Huegel, was coordinator of a practical nursing program. She received frequent requests for students to provide private duty care. There were no organized registries in our area, but a need was evident. We were commuting together and had time to discuss our ideas. I saw a unique opportunity to provide a needed service while providing flexible employment for nurses. I was interested in the business aspects and assumed responsibility for that, while my partner took charge of the clinical component. We had little competition; two firms attempted to corner our market, but we had the competitive edge.

As both nurses recognized, professional experience is a rich source of data about market needs. Pay attention to the cues, and keep asking, "Is there a market for this?"

Networking. Networking is another method of collecting information. The three components of this strategy are:

1. selection of appropriate contacts,
2. a systematic process for networking, and
3. a structured framework for active listening.

Contacts. Your purpose in networking is to keep abreast of all the issues affecting your clients and your business. Who are the people who help you meet that goal? Obviously, your clients are among them; but a number of other people also have information relevant to your business. For example, a nurse entrepreneur providing rehabilitation services to patients in their homes might develop a network that includes, but is not limited to,

- client support groups (i.e. the Multiple Sclerosis Society),
- the Home Health Care Nurses Association, and
- the Home Equipment Supply Association.

An entrepreneur's need for information is constant, but the time and energy available for pursuit of that information are limited. Targeting appropriate networks ensures that time and energy are expended efficiently and effectively. One of your early tasks in finding a niche is to build extended networks and develop a plan for interacting with people in those networks.

Systematic Networking Plan. A systematic plan for networking sustains the network and generates timely information. Networking activities include attending workshops, participating in meetings, going to conventions, and having lunch with individuals or groups. How to allocate personal resources for networking is a business decision and is based on your information goals. Therefore, these goals must be part of your planning considerations, as must the networking potential in any activity.

Use Exercise 3.4 as an aid to developing a networking plan.

✓ Exercise 3.4 Information Networking Plan.

Instructions. In the far left-hand column, list the individuals or groups that make up your potential information networks. In the next column to the right, assign a priority to each network on the basis of how important each one is as a source of information. In the third column, indicate how you intend to interact with that network (i.e. meetings, lunch). In the far right-hand column, indicate the frequency of your interactions. If possible, assign a specific date. For example, if a group holds its annual meeting in April and you want to attend, put that down.

Potential Networks	Priority	Activity	Frequency/Dates

Put this plan to work immediately to learn more about potential markets for your services. As you expand your networking activities, structure your listening to make certain that you hear all the cues.

Active listening. If you are to be an active listener, you must create a framework that enables you to attend to the information you receive in a focused way. This is accomplished by evaluating the content of any communication for

- complaints that reflect unmet or poorly met needs,
- patterns in identified problems that point to persistent problems or impending changes,
- problems of one group that might be experienced by a different group,
- indicators of systems breakdowns, and
- knowledge or skill deficits.

Deloris M. Giltner uses a varied network to keep up with the data she needs. She began a business providing psychotherapy to individuals, couples, and families as she was making the transition to retirement in 1983.

> My initial market testing included an analysis of services provided in Broomfield, CO, and the surrounding areas. I checked with ministers, schools, and the city regarding needs and relied on my experience in a gratis therapy role in my parish. I maintain contact with current and emerging client needs through church and school contacts, the input of other professionals, and review of Chamber of Commerce reports on the economy.

Literature Survey. Professional journals, newspapers, and popular magazines furnish two types of information. First, they supply data on trends, problems, and future demands. Second, they forecast changes in clients' perception of their needs. Often, journal articles raise individuals' awareness of their needs from a felt to a real level. Therefore, reading what your clients read increases the possibility that you will be among the first to recognize and act on a new market trend.

Developing a reading plan is as crucial as developing a networking plan. Make your reading time count by deciding now what to read and when to read. As you review the literature look for

- existing problems,
- advances in knowledge and technology,

- demographic changes, and
- changes in the policies, rules, and regulations formulated by political and professional regulatory bodies.

Effective data gathering is the necessary basis for any comprehensive understanding of the internal and external pressure creating client problems. Whether your clients are patients, health professionals, organizations, or any combination of these, there are two questions you must ask yourself. First, am I getting all the information possible? Second, if I am not, how can I extend my data-gathering efforts? Acquiring necessary information is the first step in a market-service analysis. The next step is to analyze that information and identify problems.

Problem Identification

Six catalysts create the types of problems that are opportunities for entrepreneurial interventions:

- challenges to expectations and values,
- organizational mandates,
- system dysfunction,
- knowledge and skill deficits,
- demographic changes, and
- professional/political/regulatory body policies.

Evaluating the data you collect within the framework of these catalysts permits precise identification of client problems.

Expectations and Values. When expectations and values are challenged, people experience problems as they attempt to alter behaviors to meet new expectations, reduce or eliminate problems associated with change, or preserve critical values.

Recent events in health care that have precipitated questioning of values and expectations include a societal interest in wellness; an emphasis on cost-versus-quality analysis in provider organizations; a drive for nursing independence; and moral-ethical dilemmas, such as ensuring access to health care for everyone. Entrepreneurs recognize the point at which attempts to balance the pressures for change and stability create new problems for clients. Understanding the role that expectations and values play in this balancing process contributes to an accurate definition of client-centered needs and opportunities for nurse interventions. Salle McDaniel describes a range of expectations and values that provided a unique business opportunity for her. In 1984, Delaware Nursing Centers, Inc., incorporated in response to the needs of a specific community.

> Community leaders desired improved access to health care for low-income people at the same time that the updated Nursing Practice Act allowed nurses to function more independently. I had a desire to improve the access to health care in this area. My response to this opportunity was to start the only nurse-managed community health center in Delaware; the only place where comprehensive primary health care is available to everyone, regardless of ability to pay. Our goals include: develop a bilingual Spanish-English staff, establish a nurse-managed primary health-care center, provide a cross-cultural training location for nurses in Delaware, develop an awareness of nursing as a viable career choice for Hispanics and other ethnic minorities, and provide a clinical site for nursing research. We hope to open the Westside Health Service to meet these goals in fall 1987.

Delaware Nursing Centers, Inc., represents a value-driven business initiated in response to needs that arose from a blend of societal, cultural, and professional values.

Organizational Mandates. Organizations possess dynamic cultures and systems that are constantly in flux. Problems emerge as organizations change direction and mobilize human, financial, and technical resources to meet new goals. When your client is an organization, your services enhance the changing relationships among four elements: human, technical, financial, and organizational. Nikki Brierton is an organizational and management development consultant. In this role, she helps organizations to coordinate these four elements successfully.

> As an assistant director for continuing education, it was apparent to me that nurses lacked training for leadership roles and that this cost the organization money, frustrated nurse managers, and decreased the credibility of nursing in the organization. As an entrepreneur, I can assist nursing departments and individual nurses adapt to and manage organizational change, develop interdepartmental relationships, intitiate work redesigns, and build management teams for operating efficiently and problem solving.

When the mandate of provider organizations conflicts with the goals of the users, enrepreneurial interventions are aimed at improving that aspect of the care delivery system. Janice Crist, of SCE Self Care Education, recognized the gap between user goals and provider organizations.

> As an RN for 13 years, I saw the effect of the health-care system ignoring the client's need for information and understanding. I decided to help

providers offer patient education by consulting with health-care agencies about patient education systems, teaching other nurses patient education skills, and providing direct patient education myself on an outpatient basis. I have increased the quality of patient education by teaching nurses how to assess learning readiness and how to streamline and individualize their teaching.

System Dysfunction. A system is a series of interdependent activities or interactions essential for achieving a desired outcome. Systems can be made up of either human or technical components, or a combination of the two. Health care comprises many subsystems, among which are care delivery, transport, staffing, acuity assessment, information gathering, equipment procurement, and reimbursement. Because of the interdependence of the components of a system, failure in even one component affects the functional ability of the whole system. Dysfunctional systems create user problems, cause frustration, increase cost, reduce quality, and make desired outcomes unattainable.

Nurses constantly invent, modify, repair, or refine systems to increase their efficiency, effectiveness, or safety. How many times have you altered some aspect of a care delivery process to obtain better results for patients? How often have you modified equipment so that it worked more efficiently? What systems have you routinely improved or enhanced to meet patient or organizational goals more readily?

Entrepreneurial nurses can use systems expertise in a variety of ways. For example, Eisenhauer (1980) describes a role for nurses in expediting user choices of health-care delivery systems. Pointing out that "a number of changes within the health-care delivery system and within society have brought about a consumer need for help in both choosing among health-care options and in obtaining health information" (p. 417), she envisions nurses as health care brokers.

Handling system dysfunctions involves knowing how to analyze systems by breaking them down into their component parts, isolate the points at which the system functions poorly, and market the services that will eliminate obstacles to achieving desired outcomes. Margaret O'Brien, of Margaret Y. O'Brien, Inc.—Health Care Consultants, brings a systems expertise to organizations for which she consults. She works with Home Health Agencies, HMOs, public health departments, community agencies, and individuals. As her brochure states, she helps them to learn "how to manage alternative healthcare that works."

My services include: in-depth market research, solid strategic planning, Medicare/Medicaid guidance, human resource development, ongoing program support, and ensured growth potential. In one organization, I was asked by the administrator and board of directors to review the

> operations of the Home Health Agency prior to determining whether or not to close down that function. My analysis proved that the agency was viable but underfinanced. As a result, more resources were allocated to the division, and it has become a viable cost center.

Knowledge and Skill Deficits. Advances in knowledge and technology present problems for both individuals and organizations. Updated knowledge and skills are necessary for remaining competitive, whether this involves developing new systems or improving old ones. Dominick S. Cullen, of CAI Management Systems, fills a special knowledge gap in organizations.

> I had an in-depth knowledge of computers and 28 years of nursing experience, much of it in management positions. I was aware of the need for computerized staffing studies and started doing this. Later, I expanded into other computer-related management projects. One of the disadvantages I face is the need to continuously seek new clients. I use creative marketing and networking to deal with this problem. An unexpected result of my networking efforts was a business inquiry from a prospective client in the Philippines—from "word of mouth" advertising.

Networking helps you to evaluate breakthroughs in knowledge and technology as sources of problems for your clients, as well as to develop services that assist them with needed changes.

Demographic Data. Population shifts or changes in the vital statistics of client populations can indicate impending problems within a particular environment. An aging population, for example, creates demands for different kinds of services, places unique requirements on provider organizations, and necessitates development of new expertise on the part of caregivers. The response Janet Moll and Delores Alford made to demographic trends resulted in the establishment of two businesses.

> In 1974, Nursing Associates was formed to provide primary health care, focusing on wellness, through health assessment, teaching, and counseling. Our clients are adults of all ages, although we focus on the elderly. We felt the public needed direct access to nurses and nurses' unique knowledge. We wanted to provide care to ambulatory older adults in the community.
>
> The Institute of Gerontic Nursing was established in 1985 to provide research, education, and consultation in gerontic nursing to nurses, health care agencies, businesses, industry, churches, professional organizations, and government agencies. The Institute developed because we were providing this kind of service through Nursing Associates and wanted to pull this activity into a separate organization. Our knowledge and philosophy as nurses and specialists in gerontological nursing gives us special skills in providing care that is not available to clients in the traditional medical-illness model system.

Review demographic trends for the possible impact they will have on the varied client and provider systems operating in the settings in which you provide services.

Political and Professional Regulatory Policies. The policies, rules, regulations, or directives of various professional and political bodies precipitate broad changes and create unique problems as individuals and organizations strive to formulate appropriate responses to new standards. An obvious example is the impact that the DRG reimbursement policies are having on health care today. Patricia C. Wilson has been helping clients through the government maze since her 1982 business start-up.

> I retired from federal service in the Medicare program and realized that providers did not understand all the regulations. They needed an advocate. I interpret Medicare regulations to home health providers. My service is unique because my knowledge of federal regulations complements my clinical experience.

Two regulatory issues of special interest to nurse entrepreneurs are entry into practice and credentialing. In addition, the trend toward increased regulation of HMOs and long-term care will both resolve and create problems for clients and providers. Joan C. Warden, of J.C. Warden & Associates, assists long-term care facilities in their regulatory struggles.

> The stimulus to become an entrepreneur occurred when I was a director of nursing in a long-term care facility. After several very favorable state surveys, it was recommended that I provide consulting in this area. I found that the industry was very much in need of this kind of service. Many facilities are struggling with rapidly changing regulations. I provide a range of services to assist these agencies: quality assurance, facility surveys, reimbursement, and marketing. My services are greatly needed and used.

Since regulatory compliance frequently effects accreditation, reimbursement, or both, the entrepreneur who facilitates that process discovers a ready client market.

Client problems can spring from any one of the six catalysts described, or from a combination of several. As you gather information about clients, consideration of the six catalysts will provide insight into the nature of their problems. Complete Exercise 3.5 to identify problems that exist in your client group.

✔ Exercise 3.5 Problem Identification.

Instructions. Complete this exercise for each of the client subgroups recorded in Exercise 3.3. In the far left-hand column, list client subgroups. In the next column to the right, indicate the source of the information you have about the client's problems (experience, networking, literature). In the third column, describe the roots of the problems (challenge to expectations, etc.). In the far right-hand column, list the problems.

Clients	Information Source	Problem Root	Problem Identification
1.			
2.			
3.			

Examine your responses to this exercise. Do you have adequate information about each client? If not, how will you improve your data gathering? If you experience difficulty with problem assessment, try working with someone else. Complete this exercise for each of your potential client subgroups before you continue with the market-service analysis.

Your success in identifying problems is limited only by the quality and quantity of your data and your ability to interpret those data. It is more than likely that you will identify more problems than you could possibly handle. The third and fourth steps in the market-service analysis make up a narrowing process, in which you transform problems into client-centered needs and decide which of these needs constitute the ideal target market for your business.

Client-Centered Needs Analysis

Client needs are generated when clients feel a desire to do something about their problems. A need is the requirement for something perceived as necessary or useful. If an entrepreneur can describe a problem in words that reflect the client's perception, he or she can identify and market services that accurately match the client's needs. This client-centered approach promotes a complementary relationship between client and entrepreneur.

Connor and Davidson (1985) list seven words or phrases that are helpful tools for describing needs for services in client-centered terms:

- improve or enhance,
- protect,
- identify,
- reduce/relieve/eliminate,
- restructure,
- restore/resolve, and
- develop/install.

In virtually any problem situation, the necessary intervention or interventions can be described in terms of one or more of these. Use them as a guide in Exercise 3.6, which focuses on identifying client-related services. You may substitute words or phrases that you think are more appropriate.

✔ Exercise 3.6 Client-Centered Needs Analysis.

Instructions. Complete this exercise for each client subgroup you listed in Exercise 3.3. First, identify the client subgroup; second, list the problems that subgroup has; and third, use the Client-Centered Service Analysis form below to describe the services that you will market to that client in client-centered terms.

1. Client ______________________________

2. Problems:

3. CLIENT-CENTERED SERVICE ANALYSIS (BLANK FORM)

For ____

(service)

Your task is to identify client needs and problem situations for which your service is appropriate. For each verb or combination of verbs listed below, identify how your service applies. For example, after the word *eliminate* you might put "unnecessary forms and procedures."

a. Improve or enhance:

b. Protect:

c. Identify:

d. Reduce, relieve, or elimiate:

e. Restructure:

f. Restore or resolve:

(Form adapted from Connor & Davidson, 1985, p.15. Used with permission.)

The end product of this exhaustive analysis of clients' needs is an extensive list of services you can market. Trying to market every one of these services, however, diffuses available resources and makes marketing difficult. If you are to develop the most productive business strategies, your next step in finding a niche is to prioritize your services and select a business focus.

Client-Centered Business Focus

The objective of this final step is to select the most productive of the business opportunities uncovered in the previous exercise. To accomplish this, you need clearly identified success goals. These goals should take into account the skills you have and most want to use in your new venture, the services that would be most cost-effective to market, and, of course, your personal and financial goals. Review the goals you listed in Exercise 3.1. Revise them if necessary, then proceed to Exercise 3.7.

✔ Exercise 3.7 Selecting a Business Focus.

Instructions. First, list your goals in order of priority, with 1 indicating the most important, 2 the next most important, and so forth. This list will help you to choose the services that will constitute your business focus.

1.	6.	11.
2.	7.	12.
3.	8.	13.
4.	9.	14.
5.	10.	15.

Second, complete a service priority matrix for each of the client subgroups listed in previous exercises. In the far left-hand column, list the client subgroups. In the next column, to the right, list the services that each client needs. In the numbered columns on the right (which correspond to the numbered goals above), place a check under one or more of the numbers if you can meet the goal or goals by providing that particular service.

SERVICE PRIORITY MATRIX																
	Service	Goals														
Client	Needed	1	2	3	4	5	6	7	8	9	10	11	12	13	14	15

Third, review the matrix carefully, and select the service that represents the best business opportunity for you.

Fourth, decide what your business is and describe that business in client-centered terms by completing the following statement.

BUSINESS FOCUS

My business is providing the following kinds of services to the clients indicated.

Clients:

Services:

I am uniquely equipped to provide these services because:

With the completion of this exercise, you have taken a major step toward finding your special niche. By describing services in client-centered terms, you make the right service-to-market connection possible. Developing a business focus that integrates your special skills gives you a competitive edge over others who might be marketing to similar client groups. A well-defined business focus equips you for market testing the business venture.

MARKET TESTING

Market testing validates a market-service analysis, and the resulting feedback furnishes ideas for ongoing business development. For the new entrepreneur, market testing represents the transition from planning to action. Marketing is discussed in greater detail in a later chapter; the focus here is on how to test market a business idea.

To market an idea, it is necessary to look at the benefits of the service from the client's perspective and recognize the steps the buyer takes as he or she moves closer to the point of deciding to purchase the service. In making a sale, each party exchanges something of value.

Steps Toward Purchase

The first step a potential buyer takes is to recognize that there is a need for a particular service. To get the buyer to see that need, address it from the standpoint of perceived customer values: saving money, improving productivity, attracting more outpatients, increasing occupancy rate, attracting specialty physicians who serve populations with specific DRGs, increasing usage of facilities by present medical staff, decreasing nursing staff turnover to reduce the need for expensive orientation classes, and so forth.

The second step that the client takes toward purchasing a service is to decide that the need is important enough to address. Enhancing awareness of all the ways in which the need is interfering with goal achievement constitutes an effective strategy for increasing client awareness of the desirability of addressing the need.

The third step the client takes toward purchasing a service is to determine that his or her facility is the appropriate site for handling the problem. A delineation of the benefits of bringing experts in to conduct continuing education classes versus those of sending people out to classes, for example, might take something like the following form (Doleysh, 1986, pp. 82–83).

- **Accurate delineation of the source of the skills deficit**. Before the initiation of any in-house educational presentation, a needs assessment is conducted to determine the source of the skills deficit. Whereas performance discrepancies resulting from the skills deficiency are amenable to educational solutions, those resulting from other causes are management problems. Educational solutions would be ineffective and wasteful of the institution's resources when performance deficiencies are not due to a skill deficiency.
- **Improved productivity and cost-effectiveness in the hospital's inservice department**. The inservice staff are working at the edges of their competence when they develop presentations in which they are not experts. Having a nursing practice expert provide the classes on nurse practice skills enables the institution's inservice staff to continue working on other programs. When they use their time to develop programs for which there are recurring needs, the inservice staff becomes more productive and more cost-effective. Improvement in courses such as staff orientation, intravenous certification, and licensed practical nurse medication classes contribute to the inservice educator's sense of mastery, service, and competence. Such successes over a period of time diminish frustration, decrease absenteeism and instructor turnover, and decrease the expenses associated with the continual preparation of the same materials.
- **The achievement of institutional objectives is best accomplished through in-house educational presentations**. By definition, in-house education presentations and community-based continuing education programs have different purposes. In-house presentations are specifically designed to improve service within the institution, whereas community-based offerings are designed to improve the individual nurse's functioning, regardless of the specialty interests of the institution.
- **In-house educational presentations are more likely to achieve institutional objectives, because presentations developed for a specific institution and based on a thorough needs assessment are the only ones that support and work within the institution's normative system**. Any consciously chosen program for change must become

absorbed into the everyday normative network of the organization if it is to survive as an element of the organization's culture. Presentations that violate or ignore the institution's norms cannot achieve the same degree of success.

- **Another reason institutional objectives are best accomplished through in-house educational presentations has to do with the number of participants likely to attend the in-house classes.** When staff members are sent to educational offerings in the community, each participant generates an additional monetary charge to the institution. The number of people sent from any one institution is usually small. When the presentation is provided in house, each additional staff member represents a per-participant decrease in the cost of providing the program. The greater the number of participants, the greater the potential for achieving and maintaining desired performance changes among staff.

The fourth step the potential client takes before becoming convinced to act is to understand how the company's service will help meet the need. If the potential client is considering continuing education classes given in-house by a clinical nurse specialist, it will be necessary to add to the information provided in the third step. The clinical nurse specialist approach is best, because it makes the needed expertise available immediately: neither time or money is wasted. It gives the client access to as much expertise as is required to solve the problem, without the long-term obligations involved in hiring an employee (pension, FICA, fringe benefits, etc.). The clinical nurse specialist expert can also implement nursing care standards, policies, and procedures, which facilitates a smooth, orderly transition in the patient care area.

The fifth step the client takes is to choose your services over those of your competitors. Document how this service will improve the institution's competitive edge. Offer to develop and implement strategies that will help the client achieve a significant return on this educational investment; as an example, you may suggest ways in which the affected service can be marketed to the client's target market to increase outpatient visits. Enumerate the advantages of working with your firm over working with your competitor's. What do you do that is unique? It might be, for instance, that all programs are based on the needs assessment; there are no "canned" programs, and every intervention is prescribed on the basis of the client's specific needs. Alternatively, it might be that your consultants are all master's-prepared nurses who fully understand the nursing care requirements of the specified patient population.

Phase 1: Research and Analysis

General Assessment. The first phase in test marketing a service is one of research and analysis, and the first step in this phase is to complete a general assessment. The general assessment is designed to give you information about the appropriateness of your idea. By the end of the assessment, you will know if there are enough potential clients to support the type of services you would like to provide, if the service has the potential to be profitable, if similar types of services have been offered successfully by other providers, and if the service you contemplate is appropriate for your company. Each part of the assessment process can be structured to culminate in a series of questions, each of which must be answered. The desirability of the service can be measured according to how many yes answers are accumulated in each set of questions. The more yes answers there are, the better the probability of success with this venture is. A no answer requires that you reevaluate your idea to eliminate the deficit you have detected.

You should be able to answer several questions after the general assessment.

- Is the service we wish to provide to hospitals, nursing homes, etc., an appropriate one for this group?
- Does our mission statement embrace the service we are considering offering?
- Does this service complement the long-range plans of this company?
- Are the financial rewards for providing this service substantial?

If the answers to all these questions are yes, you can continue with research and analysis.

Marketing Orientation. The next step in this phase of the test marketing process is to develop your marketing orientation. You must develop services that will meet your client's needs. To do that, you must make all your decisions from the perspective of your potential clients. You should identify internal resource people who are knowledgeable about marketing, and you should consider at how you can test your service before selling it to a client.

After completing this step; you should be able to answer the following questions.

- Have we examined each aspect of this service from the client's perspective?
- Does our organization possess marketing knowledge? If this is a deficit within our organization, how will we remedy this deficiency?

- Will we be able to test this service before selling it to a client? What data do we have to indicate that prior testing is or is not essential?

Identification of Potential Clients and Determination of Their Needs. The next step has two parts. You must identify potential clients (for instance, hospitals and nursing homes), and you must determine their specific needs and interests in your services. You must decide what geographic area you wish to serve, draw up a list of the appropriate institutions in that area, and survey the institutions to learn about their perceptions of the new service before it is developed.

Information Gathering. There are numerous strategies by which you can gather the information you need. One straightforward, efficient approach is to send letters informing the institutions of the service you intend to offer, and then to follow that up with a telephone call during which you obtain answers to your questions. Keep careful records of the response you get from the various places you call; you will need that information for the second phase of the test-marketing process. From the institutions that have been most helpful in answering your questions, select several to visit in person for more in-depth exploration of any further questions you have. Plan the format of that formal interview carefully, so that you can collect the most pertinent information.

Remain objective in the information collecting process. If you lead the interviewee to say what you want to hear, you risk future problems, because your response to the market will be built on inaccuracies. Be certain that the interviewee understands the purpose of your information gathering efforts. For example, you might say, "Our firm is seriously considering offering a consulting service by nurse experts on advanced critical care topics. The service is designed to focus on care and techniques pertinent to patients with complex nursing care needs who are undergoing invasive monitoring. This consulting serice would be available to your hospital on an as-needed basis. As a part of our planning process, we are talking to hospital administrators and directors of nursing to get a better idea of what you are currently doing to meet those needs that arise for expertise in nursing care that cannot be met by the people you have on staff. We are interested in knowing what some of the specific needs for expertise are in your institution and what you think about this approach to building your staff's expertise. I am not here today to sell anything, although I may be back in a few months with a specific service to offer you."

It is less threatening if you start with general needs for nursing expertise. You might begin by asking "What kinds of needs for advanced critical care nursing expertise do hospitals in this area have?" Then try to find out more about the needs this specific hospital has. Ask the interviewee what he or she thinks about the specific services you want to offer. Word the question as specifically as possible; the following questions can serve as guidelines.

- "If I were to offer to bring in a trauma clinical nurse specialist to teach your staff about military anti-shock trousers—including how to apply them, monitor them, care for the patient in them, and remove them—as well as prepare policies, procedures, quality assurance criteria, and pre- and posttests (all written specifically for your institution), would you buy it?"
- "What would have to be different about this service in order to be of interest to you?"
- "How much would you be willing to pay?"
- "Who makes the decisions here to buy this type of service?"
- Explore the acceptability of related products or services you could develop.
- "Would you be interested in purchasing a videotape that would teach your staff what they need to know to care for a multiple trauma patient in military antishock trousers?"

By the time you have conducted about a dozen of these interviews, you should be able to discern an emerging pattern of responses that will permit you to develop programs that will meet the needs of your target market. In fact, you will probably be overwhelmed by the number of needs that you have covered and could address. Accordingly, you must establish priorities in choosing what needs to address. A logical approach would be to develop the program that meets the greatest need and matches your company's capabilities to meet that need.

Having completed this step, you should be able to answer the following questions.

- Are there enough target market agencies in the area we have chosen to serve?
- Are the target market agencies interested in the service we wish to provide?
- Is there a match between the needs of our target markets and the needs our services will address?
- Have we discovered a commonality in the needs of our target market agencies?

Assessment of Own Resources. The next step involves self-assessment, with the aim of determining whether the firm possesses the specific resources necessary for providing the service you wish to offer. If weaknesses are found, you must develop a plan for overcoming them. Self-assessment should also include looking at how the firm stacks up against its competition. If a firmly entrenched competitor is already providing the service you wish to provide, a copycat approach will not be effective: Your firm must add something unique to that service. A better strategy is to try to determine whether there are any needs not being addressed by the competition that you might address.

After completing this step, you should be able to answer the following questions.

- Have we identified our strengths and weaknesses?
- Do we have sufficient expertise to build the desired service? (Other people with specific types of expertise may need to be recruited to ensure the success of the venture.)
- Do we have a competitive advantage over our competitors?
- Do we have the best chance of success with this plan?
- Have we considered the desirability and feasibility of offering to serve a need not being served by our competition?

Phase 2: Program Building

The second phase in the market testing process is that of program building. This phase includes five steps that you must go through to arrive at a program that meets the needs of the firm as well as those of the target market.

Selection. Selection of the program to be offered is the first priority. All the ideas that might have been generated are now measured against the firm's capacity to provide the right service for the right target market.

Target Marketing. By now, the target market should be fairly clearly identified, thanks in large part to the information obtained during the interviews. You have determined whether the service is more appealing to large or to small hospitals, to rural or to urban institutions, and to those with no clinical nurse specialists on the staff or to those who have clinical nurse specialists.

Design and Description of Service. You must define the service as specifically as possible. A description of the benefits the institution will realize as a result of subscribing to the service is more effective in making a sale than is a simple list of the elements of the service. Your description should include a statement of what reports, measurements, or evaluation data will be provided as a part of the service, and it should note the methods to be implemented for the purpose of monitoring the quality of the service. You must also identify the responsibilities of the client—clerical staff, xeroxing, distribution of outlines, keeping attendance lists, providing audiovisual equipment, and so forth. You should compile a list of the resources required for full development, implementation, and selling of the service as part of the program description. You should also identify what staff and services will be needed to develop the sales materials, as well as what space, equipment, materials, and staff will be necessary to deliver the program elements to the work site. Identify who will continue to serve the client by providing reports, giving evaluation, compiling measurement data or answering questions.

Costs. Costs are an essential consideration in program building. If the cost of the service is inaccurately determined, you may be faced with the prospect of going out of business or of raising prices after you have already quoted them to customers. The costs of your service must include developmental costs, staff salaries during the several months of sales activities that typically precede a sale, overhead (the cost of having and running your office), and so on. Costs include all expenses related to actual delivery of the service.

Pricing. Pricing is different from costs: it is the dollar amount you charge for providing the service. Information you obtained from the people you interviewed can be used to help establish a realistic price. Among the pricing decisions you must make is whether you will charge your clients an hourly rate, a flat fee, quarterly sums, or a set amount per participant.

After completing this step, you should be able to answer the following questions.

- Have we identified a program to develop that meets the needs of the firm as well as the needs of our target market?
- Do we possess the specific expertise required to develop and execute this service successfully?
- Have we clearly identified all characteristics of our target market?
- Have we designed and described program elements as completely as possible?
- Have we included all pertinent costs in our projections?
- Have we established a price or a price range for the service?

Phase 3: Market-Oriented Sales Plan

Process. The third phase in the process of test marketing a service is to develop a market-oriented sales plan. The first step to be considered in this phase is the process by which sales will be made. Some approaches are more effective than others in generating sales. Consider the nature of the service when determining the approach to use. Among the possible sales strategies are having a salesperson present the concept to the potential client, placing ads in newspapers or magazines, using direct mail to bring your message to the potential client's attention, renting booths at conventions, and providing seminars.

Sales Plan. Although the sales plan for a new service is often pure guesswork, it nonetheless must be written; it can always be altered after you have gained some experience in selling. The written plan should include a list of the hospitals that appear to be interested in the service along with a second list containing the names of potential clients whose interest is not known. You must determine how these hospitals will be contacted, how much time will be required to explain the service, how much time it will take to contact and see everyone on your lists, and how much time it will take to close the sale after the initial contact.

At this point, you should try to estimate the number of buyers for the service. A complex service will require more time to sell, and the ratio of calls to purchases may be lower.

Forecasting. Forecasting is the final step of sales planning. The purpose of forecasting is to build a financial statement that includes anticipated revenue and operating expenses. A basic profit-and-loss statement, measuring the forecast of sales against the costs of developing, selling, and operating the program, can be used to determine whether there will be a profit and when that profit will be apparent. Develop an operating statement for the first three years; estimate when the first sale will occur, how much revenue it will generate, and when subsequent sales will occur. In this way, you begin to build the revenue portion of the statement.

The three kinds of expenses that must be accounted for are program development, program operation, and sales. Developmental costs include such expenses as payroll, capital expense items, and supplies; they will be heaviest at the beginning. Operating costs include both fixed and variable expenses, such as payroll, facility costs (utilities and rent), maintenance, materials, publications, supplies, and travel. Sales costs include such expenses as printed and audiovisual promotional materials, payroll, travel, and postage. The forecast is revised as cost information become available. This helps to determine whether a service has been properly priced.

At this point, you must decide how long the business can survive without breaking even or making a profit. Review the forecast, and build objective criteria into your plan by which the occurrence of success or failure will be judged.

After completing this step, you should be able to answer the following questions.

- Has a process for selling the service been selected?
- Do we have a plan for contacting customers?
- Do we have a financial forecast statement that includes profits and expenses?
- Will we support the business until it becomes profitable?
- Have we developed the criteria by which the business will be judged to be a success or a failure?

Phase 4: Program Development, Evaluation, and Testing

The last phase in the test-marketing process is that of program development, evaluation, and testing. It is in this phase that monetary and other resources are committed to developing the service to the point where it can be tested. The information obtained from full development of the service provides a basis for determining its worth. This phase gives you data that can be used to assure the prospective client that the service gets results; it also gives you the opportunity to correct problems and difficulties before offering the service.

After completing this phase, you should be able to answer the following questions.

- Have we fully developed all components of the service?
- Have we proved that the service is effective, that is, that it gets results?
- Have we worked out a method by which the service can be pilot-tested?
- Have we addressed any problems that surfaced in our testing process?

Product Testing Format. If you are test-marketing a product, there are four additional steps to consider. First, you must develop a prototype of the product to show to clients. If the cost of producing the prototype is prohibitive, a drawing with a comprehensive written description will suffice. Second, you must design packaging for the product or have it designed, and the cost of packaging must be included in overhead cost calculations. Third, you must locate distributors for the product if you will not be distributing it yourself. Fourth, you must take pains to look for the most cost-effective methods of producing or purchasing the product, as well as the most cost-effective methods of delivering and storing supplies.

Inexpensive Methods for Market Testing

There are three strategies for market testing that are both effective and fairly inexpensive: space advertising, direct mail, and use of distributors.

Space Advertising. Space advertising consists of placing advertisements in regional editions of magazines and newspapers. You can often determine which magazines or newspapers will help you to get the response you want simply by looking at the number of mail-order ads the publication runs. A large number of ads suggests that others have advertised successfully in the publication.

If space advertising is to be effective, the ad must meet two criteria. First, it must be large enough: one fourth of a page is considered the minimally effective size. Second, it must contain four elements: (1) a block of text, (2) a picture, (3) a caption, and (4) an order form (Mancuso, 1987, p. 6).

The text describes your product or service. Most magazines and newspapers will help you write the ad, for a small fee. The text of the ad describes the benefits the buyer will gain from purchasing what you have to sell. An effective way of listing the benefits is to use the descriptive words that appeal to the customer's values. The following are some of the descriptive words and phrases that are most likely to induce customers to spend money.

- Money-back guarantee
- Best value for the money
- No money down, X months to pay
- Six easy payments of only X per month
- Lets you do X like an expert
- Makes your job easier, faster
- Over 20 million sold
- Act now to take advantage of this special price
- More effective, easy to operate
- Won't rust, never needs servicing
- Free 30-day trial period
- Buy two, get one free
- Automatic, foolproof, easy to clean
- Free gift if you act now
- Relax!
- Save time, save money

The picture must show the benefits the client will receive by buying your product or service. The caption under the picture is where your strongest sales pitch should be located. Your order form will be most effective if you include an 800 telephone number as well as an address.

Direct Mail. Direct mail is another effective, inexpensive strategy for testing the acceptability of your product/service. List brokers sell specialty lists that contain the names of people who are most likely to buy what you have to sell. If your concept is highly specialized, you can often rent membership lists from clubs, associations, and magazines. Your top competitors may even rent out the lists of the names of their clients.

The direct mail appeal can be put together very simply. Start with a one-page letter describing the benefits of your product/service in client-centered terms. Enclose a brochure if you want to give the client additional information about your company. If you have placed ads in magazines or newspapers, include copies of them in the direct mail package. If you have reason to believe that the recipient of your letter is actively looking for the type of service/product you are selling, you may wish to enclose something that further establishes your credibility in that area, such as a copy of an article you have had published.

In a general direct mail campaign, it is a good idea to enclose a self-addressed business envelope. Some authorities believe that providing the postage for the return envelope greatly increases the response to your mailing (Mancuso, 1987, p. 6).

If you are using direct mail to contact someone whom you believe is actively seeking a product/service that you can provide, you may wish to phone that person a few days after sending the packet in order to establish a more personal relationship and move the prospect to consider purchasing your wares. Alternatively, you can ask the person to call you (see Figure 3.6).

Use of Distributors. If you have a product to sell, you may be able to create a demand for it by making it available to distributors. To find distributors for your product, you must find retailers that handle products similar to yours and ask them which distributors they use.

In other situations, it may be appropriate to contact independent retailers to get your product into the market place. Independent retailers are entrepreneurs, too, and you should be able to convince at least a few of them to permit you to put a display in their store. If you do not charge them for the product, they have a bigger incentive to cooperate with your market testing strategy. This strategy will give you information about how you can expect your product to sell in comparison to other similar products already in the marketplace.

Now that we have considered a variety of market testing strategies, it is time to consolidate the information into an action plan. You are ready to

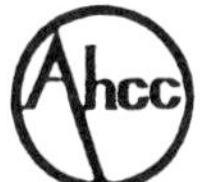

ADVANCED HEALTH CARE CONCEPTS

3799 TURNWOOD DRIVE, RICHFIELD, WISCONSIN 53076

Now you can easily *increase the quality--and cost-effectiveness--* of your nursing staff.

It starts with one quick phone call.

INTRODUCING ADVANCED HEALTH CARE CONCEPTS--YOUR ''AS NEEDED'' EXPERT CONSULTING SERVICE FOR VIRTUALLY ALL AREAS OF NURSING PRACTICE.

Give me one quick phone call and we can discuss--at no obligation--your specific needs for consulting and/or nursing education.
You can select from our unusually wide range of expertise in virtually any area of nursing practice, to accomplish goals such as

- development of ability to provide nursing care to health care markets not previously served by your institution;
- ability to care for the sicker patients you already serve with improved nursing efficiency, safety, cost-effectiveness, and confidence;
- quick and painless adoption of the utilization of new methods, knowledge, techniques, and equipment to maintain your competitive edge;
- improved ability to market your institution to prospective medical staff, thanks to superior quality of nursing staff;
- improved ability to attract and retain nursing staff;
- and much more.

All of our nurse-consultants hold master's degrees within their specialties, and all maintain clinical practices to ensure their skills and knowledge are always up to date.
Right from the start, you'll see a *marked increase in the quality* of your staff's nursing care.
What's more, you'll see a significant improvement *in your facility's bottom line*. Because an essential part of our service is to put in place many time-saving and money-saving methods that will assure you a *surprisingly quick return on your investment*.
Please look through the brochure and article reprint I've included. You'll see how we work and how we've achieved these important goals for other clients.
Then why not make that phone call? I'm at (414) 628-0251. All it takes is a few minutes of your time, and you could dramatically improve the quality of your staff--and its cost-effectiveness as well.

Sincerely yours,

Nancy Doleysh, RN, MSN
President, Advanced Health Care Concepts

P.S. Because every nursing staff is unique, I personally assure you a custom-designed program that will satisfy your specific needs. Do call, and let's talk.

Figure 3.6 Sample letter sent to prospective client.

select, test market, and provide services to clients on a trial basis. It is time to launch a trial ballon.

LAUNCHING A TRIAL BALLOON

Launching a trial balloon necessarily involves some personal risk. With each trial balloon, there is a risk that your services will be rejected. If this happens, you should not be overly upset. You gain confidence with each trial; if you experience failure, you must learn from it and launch another balloon. The previous planning exercises increase the chances for success in this trial venture. Exercise 3.8 incorporates your prior planning decisions and has as its objective the start of an actual business venture.

✔ Exercise 3.8 Launching a Trial Balloon.

Instructions. Select a service that you will market test within the next eight weeks and the client group to whom you will market this service. Complete each of the following sections.

1. The service I will market is (list in client-centered terms):

2. My target client target group is:

3. My market testing plan is:

Marketing Goal	Strategy	Action Date	Evaluation Date

4. I will evaluate the results as follows.
   a. Marketing strategy:

Strategy Utilized	Success			Comment
	Yes	No	Partial	

   b. Information: On the basis of your response to market testing,
      (1) How well was your service or product idea received?

      (2) What are clients willing to pay for this service or product?

      (3) Are you willing to begin your business with this service or product?

      (4) What is your potential market share?

5. I will take the following steps to get my business off the ground:

6. My future trial balloons—to be launched after I have a chance to learn from this trial—are:

The purpose of a trial balloon is to test the market and yourself. Perhaps your first effort will result in rapid business growth; perhaps your start will be slower. In either case, the process of finding a niche, of which launching a trial balloon is the culmination, is one that can be applied at any stage of growth.

SELF-HELP TIPS

At the beginning of this chapter, we mentioned additional strategies that may help you to find your niche: *s*eriousness, exclusivity, *l*ocation, *f*lexibility, *h*ealth and *h*umor, expertise, *l*ooks, and *p*lanning. We present these eight self-help tips here, because they are essential components of a successful business. These tips are a composite of advice from us and advice from the nurse entrepreneurs who contributed to this book.

Seriousness

Take your business seriously. Devote time and energy to its survival, limit interruptions to business time, and pursue your goals and determination. Most of all, refer to what you do as a business, not a hobby or something you are doing to keep from being bored. Think in business terms about product line, finances, contracts, and, most of all, fees. How you think about your activities will influence your behavior and convince others that you are a businessperson. You cannot find a niche without a strong belief in the validity of your enterprise.

Exclusivity

Direct your efforts toward those services and activities that are most likely to ensure success. Identify your product line, and put your energies into providing it with all the expertise you can develop. Do not attempt to pursue every option: you will fragment your efforts, and your product quality will probably decline. Market your exclusiveness—those unique skills that make you stand out from the competition. A sense of exclusivity helps you keep your eye on the bouncing ball, a necessary task if you want to stay in the game.

Location

Find space for your business, whether that space is a rented office or a corner in your home. Work effectiveness, time management, and your sense of a business self depend upon an appropriate work environment. This is especially important if clients come to you, because image is involved. Locating a space with a purely business function eliminates the need to keep moving papers and materials, improves record-keeping accuracy, and contributes to consistent work patterns.

Flexibility

Although this tip may appear to contradict the second tip, they are actually two ends of a single continuum. Flexibility implies staying in touch with the client milieu, constantly assessing emerging problems, and developing new services when good business sense dictates. Flexibility will prevent you from staying emotionally tied to a service or product even when clients' needs have changed. Instead, it will ensure that you maintain a competitive edge in your business.

Health and Humor

Take care of yourself. Learn to recognize stress signals, and take time out for relaxation and exercise. Learn to laugh at and with yourself. Entrepreneuring demands stamina and commitment and frequently places you in stressful situations. Developing your physical and mental coping ability will help you maintain the level of wellness you need to enjoy your success.

Expertise

Remember that clients are paying for your professional expertise, and use strategies to avoid obsolescence (such as reading, workshops, or maintaining a client practice). When certain aspects of your business demand expertise you do not have, make use of the expertise of others. A marketing consultant may make a difference in how your business grows. You may subcontract a portion of a consulting project to another professional with a unique service to offer. The important point is to recognize the need for expertise and know how to develop it in yourself or locate others who have the needed skills.

Looks

Create an image for yourself and your business. Your image and the style with which you present yourself and your business send a message to clients about such qualities as competency, credibility, and organization. Consider the image you project when you dress or speak. Evaluate your nonverbal behaviors, and proofread material going out under your business name. When you and your business are "looking good," your heightened self-esteem increases your personal effectiveness.

Planning

Planning is the sine que non of any successful business. It not only helps you find a niche but ensures that you will stay in that niche. It is a constant activity: staying in business necessitates commitment to a process of continued formal planning. Decide now on a planning timetable. During planning time, review goals, do a market service analysis, revise goals, and develop action steps and timeliness. Planning will enable you to recognize and pursue optimal business opportunities.

In the last three chapters, you have moved from inquiry to action on the entrepreneurial career path. You have found a niche. With the launching of a trial balloon, you will initiate activities that will result in the emergence of a business. The work of the previous chapters lays a business foundation. In part II, we will provide the building materials you need to develop that business.

II ESTABLISHING A BUSINESS: READY, SET, GROW

In this section, we introduce you to the business side of entrepreneurship. Chapter 4 shows you how to write a business plan and how to find the resources you need as you start a business. Chapters 5, 6, and 7 explain in greater detail the organizing, marketing, and financing components of a business and of business planning. Chapter 8 takes you beyond the start-up period to a consideration of the issues of survival and growth.

4 PLANNING A NEW BUSINESS

The transition from testing a business idea to developing a successful enterprise is challenging, exciting, rewarding, and filled with the nitty-gritty details that constitute serious planning. According to one source (*The New Business Guide*, 1986), "most successful entrepreneurs spend at least six to ten months researching and preparing their ventures." A well-planned business start-up makes the difference between success and early failure (or, at best, painfully slow growth). As Merril and Sedgwick (1987) remark, "the day you open your door, the clock starts running. If you don't know what you're doing, it's too late to learn. If you don't have a plan, it's too late to figure one out" (p. 5). For this reason, we explore the process of developing a business plan and reviewing the research and resources that assist in that task now, before addressing questions of organization, marketing, and finance. In what follows, we pay particular attention to those trends and issues that specifically affect nurse-run businesses.

THE BUSINESS PLAN

Formulating a business plan is the most effective method for addressing all the contingencies that face the entrepreneur perparing to start a business. The thorough analysis needed to complete a business plan increases the chances for business success in the following three ways:

1. The plan addresses decisions that you should make before engaging in the day-to-day routine of running a business. The comprehensive understanding of the nature of your business that you will gain from developing a plan helps you answer certain crucial questions: How should I approach potential customers? How much should I charge to make a profit? Do I need a partner?
2. Developing a plan helps you anticipate business decisions. Your planning projections will keep you on course, or point out when you are in trouble with respect to specific components of the business, such as financing, potential sales, or profits.

3. The plan interests others in providing needed financing, because it demonstrates that you command in-depth knowledge of the business, its potential, its financial needs, and its ability to provide an excellent return on the investor's capital.

Components of a Business Plan

The business plan typically contains the following 17 components (Kelley, 1981, pp. 45–46).

1. Cover page. This includes the name, address, and phone number of the company; the date; and the names of the principals.
2. Executive summary. This is a one- or two-page explanation of the major features of your proposal.
3. Table of contents. The major sections of this component have to do with (1) the business, (2) financial data, and (3) supporting documents. Topics and page numbers are listed in the table of contents.
4. Description of your company. This explains what business you are in and what services you provide.
5. Survey of the industry. This describes the history, present state and future prospects of the industry in which you have positioned yourself.
6. Market research and analysis. This section describes your competition, the size of your market, and trends in the industry. It identifies your customers, your estimated market share, and your projected sales.
7. Marketing plan. This section explains how you intend to reach your prospective clients.
8. Management team. This section should contain an organizational chart and a job description for managers. Include a description of management, ownership, and compensation policies, and identify the board of directors, if appropriate.
9. Supporting professional assistance. List the attorneys, accountants, bankers, insurance agents, and other professionals whose services you have used to extend your management skills.
10. Operations plan. This section describes how and where you will carry out your major business activity.

11. Research and development. This section describes improvements you intend to make in your service/product or your business process. It also addresses development of new services or products.
12. Overall schedule. This section presents the timeline you will implement for all major events important to starting and developing your business.
13. Critical risks and problems. This section covers internal and external threats to the business—for instance, unfavorable trends in the industry, strong responses from your competitors, or inability to achieve sales projections.
14. Financial plan. This section presents financial forecasts and projections for the first three years.
15. Proposed financing of the company. After determining the financial needs of the company, it is necessary to determine the specific sources which will provide the financing. This section lists those sources.
16. Legal structure of the company. Sole proprietorship, partnership, and corporation are the three most common legal structures.
17. Appendices/supporting documents. This section includes any additional documents you may need to bolster your overall presentation.

Executive Summary. The executive summary is written after the rest of the plan has been completed. It should briefly describe the most important aspects of your plan: your intended clients, your current and planned services/products, the unique features and competitive advantages of these services/products, sales and profit projections, your financing needs, and the projected return on the investor's equity.

The summary will be affected by your purpose in writing the plan. Plans may be written to serve as working documents for day-to-day business decisions, or to attract outside investors. Different versions of the same plan may be prepared to meet the varied requirements that the plan must satisfy.

Table of Contents. The table of contents enables the reader to quickly determine what is included in the plan and where it is located. Different readers are interested in different aspects of the plan; a table of contents saves them time. One strategy for increasing the probability that a venture capitalist will read beyond the summary is to include illustrations, tables, and graphs in the table of contents. Six or so additions of this type will stimulate the reader's curiosity, whet his or her appetite for more information, and encourage further exploration of your plan.

Description of Your Company. Here you should describe how and why you started the business (or will start the business), the services you offer, and who your customers are. Explain how your company has progressed so far and how you differ from your competitors. Indicate the effect of new technologies on your business: what new markets will open up, and how you intend to take advantage of them. Include projections of where you think the company will go in the next ten years.

Survey of the Industry. Include a short history of the industry you are entering and a description of the major developments that shaped it. Discuss the present status of the industry, including services/products, markets, and dominant firms. Consider trends in the industry, and examine internal and external phenomena as sources of trends. An internal trend could be a new service/product developed by your company. External trends occur in the entire milieu outside of the company. They may take the form of demographic changes, new government regulations, or changes in customer demand. The sources you used in arriving at your projections should be identified.

Market Research and Analysis. This is the part of the plan that is written first. Obtain data supporting the conclusion that a market exists for your service/product (see chapter 3). These data may come from trade associations, government reports, published material, marketing research firms, hospital associations, medical societies, nursing organizations, nursing schools, or the local Chamber of Commerce. Determine the size of your market, then identify the trends in that market. Project the extent of your market penetration initially, after one year, after three years, after five years, and after ten years.

Assess your competitors, noting their size, patrons, product, price, performance, profitability, weaknesses, and strengths. Determine whether their business is increasing or decreasing and what their market share is. Anticipate the response your competitors will make to your service/product.

Using your market research, analyze your market. Identify your clients, estimate your potential annual sales to each, and assess your potential market share. Estimate your market share for each quarter over the next three years. Consider the size, trends, and growth rate of the market, as well as the growth rate of the competition. Determine your standing in the marketplace in relation to your competitors. Indicate whether your market position will improve over time.

Carefully note the characteristics of your clients, and group them according to these characteristics. Learn all you can about your potential clients, since this information will be necessary if you are to develop an effective marketing campaign.

Estimate your potential sales to each client. Be aware of the assumptions that you are making in determining your estimates, and keep your assumptions realistic.

Marketing Plan. This is the second part of the plan to be written. The strategies you will use to reach your target market must be developed and described, with attention paid both to what will be done and to who will do it. The optimal marketing approach varies according to the nature of the particular client you wish to attract. You may wish to emphasize results, price, service, or experience, depending on the specific characteristics of each market group. That decision must be made, and your marketing materials must be based on the decision.

Your plan must also address how you will reach your potential customers. Will you use salespeople, direct mail, ads in newspapers and magazines, or booths at trade conventions? Determine how much these activities will cost and how long you can afford to continue engaging in them without generating a profit.

Management Team. There are numerous functions that must be performed in any business: marketing, planning, accounting, financing, and a host of others. In a sole proprietorship, the owner performs all functions. A management team increases the likelihood of success, particularly if key managers are chosen because they possess abilities that complement the abilities of the entrepreneur.

Include succinct versions of your management team's resumes that stress the training, experience, and accomplishments of each manager; more complete resumes are traditionally included in the appendix. Correlate the manager's abilities to his or her duties in the company.

Include an organizational chart and a job description for each manager's position. List the compensation that each manager will receive. Be sure to mention ownership privileges, if you will be offering them as a form of compensation for significant performance or as a trade-off benefit in lieu of salary.

A board of directors is appropriate if your company incorporates. Remember to choose directors to complement the expertise of the entrepreneur and the management team.

Supporting Professional Assistance. Accountants, lawyers, bankers, and insurance agents are essential to any business start-up: they extend the entrepreneur's expertise in a cost-effective manner. Choose these experts for the expertise they can bring to the building of your business.

Operations Plan. This part of the plan describes how the work will get done. It describes your personnel, equipment, and office/manufacturing needs. It outlines the process by which your service or product will be produced, showing who does what, how much time is required for each step in the process, and how much each step costs.

Research and Development Program. This section details the amount of money to be spent on research and development. In a start-up, research and development costs can be projected as a percentage from financial data.

This percentage can then be compared to the percentage your competitors spend on research and development.

Overall Schedule. This section covers the major milestones in the progress of the business: when it will open, when you will begin your sales campaign, when you will see your first customer, and when the first payment will be received. Prepare a month-by-month schedule to show that activities will be done and how they will help you reach your goals. Since all activities take longer than anticipated, build additional time into the schedule. Plan for an activity to take 50 to 100 percent more time than you think it should (Kelley, 1981, p. 55).

Critical Risks and Problems. Critical problems arise as a result of both internal and external events. An example of a critical problem of internal origin would be prolonged illness of the entrepreneur. Examples of external risks or problems for a business with a clinical focus would be restrictive nurse practice acts, the high cost of malpractice insurance, or a competitor's actions. One particularly unfavorable trend in the health-care industry is increasing law suits involving nurses. Having identified critical risks and problems, describe how you would cope with them if they should arise and how you would minimize any negative impact they might have on the business.

Financial Plan. This is the third part of the business plan to be written. In this section, all your plans are translated into dollars and cents. The five documents essential to the financial plan are (1) the balance sheet, (2) the cash-flow projection, (3) the break-even analysis, (4) the income (or profit-and-loss) statement, and (5) the budget deviation analysis.

The balance sheet summarizes your company's assets and liabilities. By subtracting the liabilities from the assets, you identify your company's net worth. The balance sheet is prepared (1) for the start-up period, (2) semi-annually for the first year, and (3) at the end of each of the first three years of operation.

The cash-flow projection describes the amounts and types of cost disbursements and receipts. It tells you how well cash is being managed. A positive balance is referred to as the company's liquidity. Cash-flow projections are prepared for a three-year period. The first year's projections are done on a month-by-month basis.

The break-even analysis shows the amount of revenue needed to cover all costs. This amount is known as the break-even point. If your sales projections fall short, you may have to find some way to lower the break-even point. Describe how you could do that if necessary.

The income (or profit-and-loss) statement is developed with the help of information from other parts of your business plan. Using the information from the sales forecast, you can determine how much money you will have to work with. You can then subtract costs listed in the operations plan from your projected sales revenue to arrive at your profitability.

The budget deviation analysis is a calculation that ensures that you stay within the parameters of your budget. Performing this analysis monthly enables you to notice deviations quickly and puts you in a position to remedy negative deviations and to capitalize on positive deviations. Experience will quickly show you which budget figures should be assessed for deviation.

Proposed Financing. Describe your sources of financing. Entrepreneurs usually live off their savings, a spouse's salary, and money obtained from friends and relatives. If outside financing is necessary, you must determine which sources are most appropriate for your purposes. Your business plan details the source of the money, the amount obtained, and the purposes for which the money will be used.

Legal Structure. There are advantages and disadvantages to each of the various forms of business structure (see chapter 5). Do not settle on the form of your business until you have discussed it with your accountant, your attorney, or both. They can point out the advantages and disadvantages of each form and help you choose the form most appropriate to your particular situation.

Appendices. Supporting data may include resumes of key personnel; personal financial requirements and statements; publications by key personnel; significant letters of reference; copies of leases, contracts, and legal documents; and newspapers, magazines, or books related to the business, the industry, or your competitors.

These components make up the typical format of a business plan. If your business has unique aspects, you may want to provide additional depth or complexity or utilize alternative categories not ordinarily seen in a start-up business plan. Entire books have been written on the topic; any assistance you need beyond these basic considerations may be obtained from them.

Be thorough in preparing your business plan, but avoid unnecessary complexity—a powerful temptation for many new entrepreneurs. Remember this advice: "Concentrate on conveying the unique value of your company, and you can write a superb business plan the first time, without copying anyone else's format" (Merril & Sedgwick, 1987, p. 280).

The checklist of common business plan deficiencies in Table 4.1 will help you to avoid other pitfalls.

TABLE 4.1 Common Business Plan Deficiencies

Hype of any sort
No table of contents
No executive summary

TABLE 4.1 (cont.)

Executive summary fails to summarize
Executive summary is too long (more than ten sentences or two pages is too long)
Business plan is too short (less than 10 double-spaced pages is too short)
Business plans is too long (more then 30 double-spaced pages is currently considered too long)
Plan fails to say what the customer has to gain
Plan fails to say what the investor has to gain
No market research
No description of specific market strategy
Excessive fixation on product
No consideration of production costs
Founding team is not adequately described
No historical financial records (if company is not start-up)
No financial projections
Financial projections are too skimpy (e.g., broken down only by year, or lacking detailed expense breakdown)
Sales projections are drawn from thin air
No cash-flow projection
No balance-sheet projection
No consideration of possible problems
Projections are incompatible with standard ratios of the industry, and no explanation is given for deviation
Plan does not present proposed deal specifically (what do you want from the investor, for what?)
No discussion of proposed use of funds
Use of Funds section is vague
Company is grossly overvalued
No consideration of when and how investor can cash in
Present stock distribution and debt situation of company are not described
Plan has too may typos or sloppy grammar
Plan is shoddy in appearance, or excessively luxurious
Plan is out of date

From Merril & Sedgwick, 1987, p. 284.

The basic components of a business plan are similar for all entrepreneurs, but nurses starting their own businesses face special problems during the planning stage. These problems reflect certain trends in the health-care industry that are developing as more nurses attempt to move into independent professional practices.

PLANNING ISSUES AFFECTING NURSE ENTREPRENEURS

There are four major hurdles that nurses face as they move toward independence. Nurses in private practice, especially nurse anesthetists, nurse midwives, and nurse practitioners, encounter these barriers more than other nurses do. The four hurdles are

1. restrictive nurse practice acts,
2. competitive blocks to practice,
3. inability to obtain or high cost of malpractice insurance, and
4. limitations on third-party reimbursement for nursing services.

The causes and effects of these four barriers are interrelated. Underlying causes of these problems include the difficulty the profession has had in establishing a consensus among members about a definition of nursing, a lack of understanding on the part of the public about the role and health impact of nursing care, the traditional attitude of physicians about the role of nurses, the increased competition for patients generated by a physician overload, and the historical inclusion of the costs of nursing care in the "sheets and eats" bill instead of a direct costing out of such care.

The restrictive impact of these problems on nurses in private practice can be considerable. For example, in some states, a nurse may provide psychotherapy to a patient and receive third-party reimbursement only if that care has been ordered by a psychiatrist. The practice of nurse anesthetists and nurse midwives has been curtailed by the refusal of certain hospitals to grant privileges and the increasing difficulty of obtaining professional liability coverage.

The challenges are enormous but not insurmountable. Nurses like Cynthia Casoff, CNM, director of the Downtown Women's Center in New York City, are starting and succeeding in business in spite of these problems.

> I started my business in October of 1986, and since then my malpractice insurance has risen to $4,000 annually. However, I feel that is part of doing business now that I'm playing with the big boys. There are restrictive practices: some hospitals won't allow nurse midwives on their staff. But I feel there is enough for all of us, and there are clients who

> want alternative sources of health care. These are the women who come to the nurse midwife. I practice at St. Vincent's hospital. The hospital's willingness to allow nurse midwives to practice is based on an economic motive. A few years ago, they were ready to close their maternity service because of declining census. They decided to accept nurse midwives on the staff, and this was supported by certain physicians. Today, St. Vincent's has one of the most sought-after maternity services in the city. This turnaround is due primarily to nurse midwives.

Clearly, an informed public, aware of the value of nursing as an alternative source of care and of the cost-effectiveness of that care, is an ally in nurses' struggles against practice barriers.

Barriers to practice are one part of the problem facing nurse entrepreneurs; difficulty in obtaining reimbursement for that practice is another. Nurses in private practice find reimbursement from Medicare/Medicaid next to impossible to obtain, and in many states direct third-party reimbursement for nursing care has been blocked by legislation. For these reasons, nurse entrepreneurs like Lenore Boles and Linda Hackett, partners in Nurse Counseling Group, have devoted time and energy to changing the insurance laws in their state.

> We haven't experienced competitive barriers to practice from physicians. We are well known in the health care community, and about 30 percent of our client referrals come from physicians. Third-party reimbursement has been difficult. We worked many long hours through our state nurses' association to change the insurance law in Connecticut. We have a good law today, but there are still problems with companies based outside the state: they do not have to comply with the reimbursement mandate. Forget Medicare/Medicaid—we don't get reimbursed from them.

These issues are difficult ones, but potential nurse entrepreneurs must confront them if they are to survive in business. Fortunately, there are several methods nurses can use to confront the issues.

1. Participate through your state nurses' association and specialty associations to change the Nurse Practice Act, if necessary, and to make changes in legislation regulating third-party reimbursement.
2. Work with state legislators and your professional associations to develop alternative solutions to malpractice insurance problems. For example, the Wisconsin Health Care Liability Plan provides liability insurance to professional groups for which liability insurance is not available. As we write (August 1987) the Wisconsin Nurses' Association is petitioning the Commissioner of Insurance to add nurse

practitioners to the plan. The ANA continues to work on this problem. Follow current nursing literature for information on insurance issues.

3. Contact your representative in Congress about legislative changes in Medicare/Medicaid that will support community-based nursing organizations as alternative care models and allow nurses to compete in the health-care system. You can keep informed about legislative issues by contacting the American Nurses' Association, Washington Office, 1101 Fourteenth Street, NW, Suite 200, Washington, DC 20005, (202) 789-1800; or the National League for Nursing, Office of Public Policy, 10 Columbus Circle, New York, NY 10019, (212) 582-1022.
4. Market to individual third-party payors or insurance companies. Many nurses in private practice have been able to demonstrate the cost-effectiveness of their care and obtain a referral base of clients.
5. Search for opportunities to market nursing to community groups as an alternative source of health care. Increasing the public demand for nursing services will affect legislative changes.
6. Consider legal advice if you believe you are meeting with anticompetitive practices that unfairly limit your practice.
7. For more information on this topic, review the videotape *Breaking Down The Barriers To Nursing Practice*, prepared by the National League for Nursing. For ordering information, call toll-free (800) 847-8480 or, in New York State, (800) 442-4546.

These are some of the measures taken by nurse entrepreneurs to deal with barriers to independent practice. As you develop your business plan, determine the extent to which these barriers will affect you, and decide on the actions you will take to diminish the impact they have on your business. The course of action you choose will influence the money, time, and energy demanded of you. Planning for potential hurdles before you start the business will increase your initial operating efficiency.

As should now be clear, planning is vital for business survival. Consequently, the broadest possible array of resources should be employed in formulating a plan. The following section reviews the resources available to entrepreneurs and discusses how to locate and use them effectively.

RESEARCH AND RESOURCES

Both of use believe that our initial planning paid off in helping us make smooth transition to independence. Every situation is different, but the research we did and the resources we used may offer useful guidelines for readers.

> Gerry attended a workshop, "Establishing a Consulting or Private Practice" presented by Suzanne Hall Johnson, of Hall Johnson Communications, Inc., during which she identified a business idea and selected a business name. The workshop also provided pragmatic approaches to planning a business start-up. Nancy attended a similar workshop and in addition sought advice from the Small Business Development Center at the University of Wisconsin–Extension. Both of us reviewed the literature for information about entrepreneuring and starting, financing, and marketing a business. Each of us used an attorney's advice about business structure, taxes, and contracts. Nancy's attorney discussed potential legal problems (i.e., should there be a noncompetition clause in contracts with clinical nurse specialists who subcontracted with the business?). An accountant helped to set up the books for Advanced Health Care Concepts. His suggestions about tax laws, record-keeping, depreciation of equipment, and state requirements were invaluable.

The process we followed included four planning activities: self-directed reading; locating public, professional, and private resources; selecting and using expert advice; and acquiring business and organizational memberships.

Self-Directed Reading

Libraries are an excellent source of information about entrepreneurship and all aspects of business development and management. Moreover, they frequently publish or display information about community agencies that provide assistance to new businesses. Both of us found books, pamphlets, and brochures to be helpful tools during the developmental stages of our businesses. Much of your initial planning work will be done in the course of self-directed activities that help you explore options and analyze entrepreneurial possibilities.

Tapping Into Community Resources

Most communities have a variety of agencies, groups, or businesses that help the new entrepreneur. This assistance may take the form of information and advice or may include help with some or all of aspects of new business development. For illustrative purposes, we list five resources available in the Milwaukee area that exemplify the type of help you are likely to find in your community.

1. The Small Business Association provides counseling, workshops, publications, and (in certain cases) financial assistance to small businesses.

2. Each of the two major universities in the city has a unit designed to promote entrepreneurial endeavors. The University of Wisconsin, Division of Outreach and Continuing Education, has established the Business Development Center. This unit assists entrepreneurs with all phases of new business development and operations, including market testing, business plan development, locating financial assistance, and selecting marketing strategies. At Marquette University, College of Business Administration, the Center for Study of Entrepreneurship is a valuable source of advice, workshops, seminars, and information for the entrepreneur.
3. The Milwaukee Innovation Center is a privately owned business that provides assessment and market analysis for new products and innovative business ideas and links entrepreneurs with potential venture capital sources.
4. The Wisconsin Nurses' Association has sponsored workshops for nurses interested in starting their own business.

In addition to the organizations that offer these general services to entrepreneurs, there are many whose services are highly specialized, such as those that focus on market testing, planning, operations management, or financial management. There are even firms whose sole purpose is to help the entrepreneur select the right business name.

To gain access to this array of helpful sources, start by calling the Small Business Association; local colleges and universities; national, state, and local professional organizations; and the local Chamber of Commerce. When you make contact, ask about

1. the type of help they provide to a new entrepreneur;
2. the cost of this help;
3. pamphlets, brochures, or other information available;
4. educational workshops, seminars, or programs planned on the topic;
5. banks and other sources of financial assistance in the community that specialize in helping new businesses;
6. other community agencies or groups that might be of assistance to you;
7. groups in the community whose members are small business owners; and
8. ways of locating professional experts; e.g., lawyers, accountants, marketing consultants, planners, and so forth.

Each contact will add to your store of information and lead to other sources of help. When you have acquired an overview of the resources available in your community, you can begin to sort through the information and use it to develop your business plan or to select professional experts who will bring skills you do not possess to the planning process.

Selecting and Using Experts

If you decide to hire an expert, there are specific strategies you should employ that will make your use of this resource more efficient.

1. Be clear about your goals for these interactions. What kind of help do you need, and what outcomes do you expect from the interaction?
2. Get an "up front" estimate of the cost of the service.
3. Clarify mutual expectations. What work will the expert do, and what part of the project will be your responsibility?
4. Find out how available the expert will be. Will you have to wait several days for an appointment when you need help?
5. Make sure there is a good personality match. If you are not satisfied, switch to a different expert.
6. Settle issues of control early. This is your business; you are seeking expert advice, but the decisions are yours to make.

The extent and type of expertise needed are different for each entrepreneur; you are the best judge of which skills will complement the strengths you have. Many entrepreneurs hesitate to use experts because they are not sure how to locate competent professionals. The best way of finding reliable experts is to network with other entrepreneurs who have used similar resources.

Joining Peer Groups

Developing contacts with other entrepreneurs at this stage is crucial. We have derived benefit from a variety of groups, especially those whose members are nurses and women. One of the community business groups to which we belong is the Wisconsin Women Entrepreneurs. In this group, we discovered an extensive network of information about the financial and political milieu of our community and how these affect women in business. Frequently, organization members have expertise we need or can direct us to someone who does. Speakers at meetings address issues relevant to entrepreneurs.

At the national level, the Nurse Consultants Association, has been an excellent support source for us (see the description in chapter 1). This and other such groups provide nurse entrepreneurs with opportunities to learn and grow and to share what they have learned with others. Find and participate in those groups of entrepreneurs whose members share your problems, concerns, and goals.

In many new businesses, the major problems and concerns are related to how to get started. There are important decisions to be made, and entrepreneurs desperately need information if they are to make those decisions properly. There is no substitute for doing your homework (research) and finding and using the best resources available. Exercise 4.1 will help you accomplish this.

✓ Exercise 4.1 Research and Resources.

Instructions. Locate the information and help you need to plan your business start-up. Begin with calls to agencies listed in part I, and continue until you believe you have discovered all the appropriate resources available to you.

I. PUBLIC AND PROFESSIONAL ORGANIZATIONS		
Agency	Information/Help Provided	Cost
Small business association		
Chamber of Commerce		
Colleges/ universities		

I. PUBLIC AND PROFESSIONAL ORGANIZATIONS		
Agency	Information/Help Provided	Cost
Professional organizations (specify)		
Others (list)		

II. PRIVATE AGENCIES		
Agency	Information/Help Provided	Cost
Banks that will work with small businesses		
Other agencies (specify)		

III. ORGANIZATIONS. List the organizations you might consider joining and indicate the amount of dues for each organization. What benefits will you derive from membership? Be as specific as possible.

Organization	Benefits	Due

IV. WORKSHOPS OR SEMINARS. List the title, sponsoring agency, date, and cost of workshops or seminars you might attend.

Title	Agency	Date	Cost

V. PLANNING ASSISTANCE REQUIRED. Review the questions in the Workcopy Business Plan Outline in Appendix 2 to determine the type of help you need to develop your business plan. List the required expertise below, and indicate the approximate cost of the assistance.

Expertise Required	Approximate Cost of Service

You have now complied a list of the resources available to you and estimated the approximate cost of developing a business plan. In addition, you can select from the plan development information at your command only those elements appropriate for you, because your unique business circumstances dictate the extent and complexity of planning necessary. A well-thought-out plan that matches your specific situation supports a smooth and successful business start-up.

5 ORGANIZING A BUSINESS START-UP

For each entrepreneur, there is a moment when the time is right to act and get the business off the ground. The purpose of the planning process detailed in chapter 4 is to prepare you to organize an efficient start-up when you reach this point. Organization is the establishment of a structured process for carrying out the myriad tasks necessary to the operation of a business in such a way that the outcome of each activity is consistent with your overall business goals. Such a process is developed through a series of decisions that determine how your business is run.

ORGANIZING DECISIONS

The key decisions that you must make to get your business up and running are listed in Table 5.1. These decisions will shape your business operations and help you to attain your personal and business goals.

Some of the items in the checklist may appear too simple to be worth worrying about. Remember, however, that an efficient operating process not only allows you to get a good start and keep up with or pass the competition, but also decreases the stress you experience. Imagine talking with your first major client and frantically trying to find a pen that writes. Sometimes the small details make a big difference. In this chapter, we will address the organizing details, small and not so small, that determine start-up efficiency.

DEVELOPING A BUSINESS PHILOSOPHY

Most nurse entrepreneurs have a clearly defined set of beliefs about nursing and nursing practice. Integrating these beliefs into an overall business philosophy influences business operations in several ways.

Generating a Code of Business Ethics

Nurses entering the business world face new moral and ethical dilemmas. A clearly defined code of business ethics will help you to resolve these

TABLE 5.1 Key Start-Up Decisions
DECISION AREAS
Identify a business philosophy
Identify business goals
Start-up
Expansion
Select the appropriate form
Sole proprietorship
Partnership
Corporation
Create the business image
Select a name for the business
Locate space
Home
Office
Identity plan
Incubator
Decide on purchased services
Secretary
Computer
Mailing
Printing
Experts: lawyer, accountant, etc.
Select equipment
Office supplies
Office furniture
Computer/typewriter
Telephone
Answering machine
Clinical practice equipment
Beepers
Design an effective work process
Time management
Communication
Team building
Evaluating
Personal–professional development
Develop an organized documentation process

problems. Joan C. Warden, president of J.C. Warden & Associates, a firm that provides consultant services for long-term care, describes how her code helps her handle a client's lack of response to interventions.

> As I enter each facility, I consider it to be my facility and work to provide the very best service possible. I will not remain with a facility unless I can see progress within the first six months. If there is no progress, I do not continue to accept fees from this client.

Nikki Brierton is another organizational consultant whose ethical code guides her interaction with clients.

> My philosophy is to respond to clients' goals and objectives that are in keeping with my ethics and morals. I cannot work with organizational double messages.

Developing a code that expresses your core business values increases your ability to deal with unexpected ethical dilemmas confidently.

Establishing a Business Orientation

Your statement of philosophy should also reflect a commitment to making sound business decisions that ensure the company's survival. Barb Dalpaz, of Moss Bay Preventive Medicine, describes how she and her partner view this commitment.

> We need to understand every aspect of the business and know where our money is. We will never just hand it over to let someone else "do the numbers". Our accounts receivable ceiling will be minimal: under $200. These business-oriented values were the basis for our start-up goals: (1) watch prices, shop for the best deals; (2) stay within a budget of $15,000; (3) use our common sense when making decisions—not other people's advice; (4) keep communication at a maximum between us.

This example demonstrates how a business-orientation affects start-up decisions and the operating processes employed.

Enhancing Client Relationships

Nurse entrepreneurs bring something special to their clients, and that something is a natural outgrowth of a specific philosophy. Lorraine Jacobson, of Wingspan, exemplifies that philosophy when she states that her goal is "to serve the client with integrity and excellence in an environment that promotes a sense of well-being." Geneie Everett Fellows, of Humanistic Programming & Planning, has specific beliefs about client participation in her work as an architectural and facilities consultant.

> I wanted to improve facilities that were built for people. My business philosophy incorporates the need to stress user involvement in building, planning, and evaluation.

Another nurse whose philosophy incorporates elements of client control and accountability is Barbara Klein, who contracts with insurance carriers to coordinate the medical rehabilitation and return to work of workers who have suffered industrial injuries or nonindustrial catastrophic injuries.

> I believe that when people are given permission and a choice, they often recover much more quickly. Because I integrate this in my practice, numerous clients have opted to take charge of their healing, to choose an optimal outcome—e.g., postsurgery recovery with remarkable speed and functional ability where this was not thought possible.

These examples illustrate the two ways in which a client-focused approach influences the business process. First, such an approach specifies the priority placed on client needs as a driving force for excellence in business; second, it classifies the expectations and roles that client and entrepreneur have in any interaction. This second influence is important in situations in which a client must assume responsibility for the outcome of any intervention, clinical or management, if that intervention is to be successful.

Creating an Organizational Climate

If your business includes others—partners, associates or employees—your philosophy will affect the overall climate of the organization. For this reason, Dianne Duchesne, executive director of Nurses In Transition, includes "attention to process-group dynamics in relationships among staff" in her business philosophy. Elizabeth Dayani, corporate administrator of American Nursing Resources Home Health Agency, Inc., has a business philosophy that integrates caring for both client and staff: "My philosophy is simply stated: The client is number one, the worker is number two. Take care of both—both client and worker need to feel cared about."

Recoginizing, and supporting the needs of work groups in your organization's value system makes team building much easier and encourages workers to make important contributions to start-up. The resulting gains in cohesiveness, morale, and productivity are crucial for organizational effectiveness.

A philosophy generates vision and values for the business. As these examples prove, developing a business philosophy need not be a complicated task: A simple statement of the beliefs and values that will guide your practice provides a useful touchstone for future decisions and actions.

GOALS AS AN ORGANIZING STRATEGY

In chapter 3, we discussed goals and provided examples of start-up goals. Like your business philosophy, you goals should be developed in order to provide direction for the activities of your new business. If you are unsure what outcomes you desire, your initial business activities may be fragmented, and your resources may be expended to little or no point. If more than one person is involved in the operation, failure to establish goal directives that everyone understands creates a chaotic business climate in which people are working at cross-purposes and success is elusive. At a later stage, your goals help you to evaluate your progress. If you are not meeting your goals, you must try to determine whether your business resources (people, time, energy, and money) are being used appropriately or whether the goals were unrealistic in the first place.

Be careful not to overcomplicate what should be a simple procedure. Developing goals basically entails asking, "What do I want to achieve through my business?" The process of goal development should facilitate action rather than impede it. Elaborate statements are not necessary, but clear, concise, realistic, and measurable terms are. The more sensible your goals, the better the chances that all your business activities will result in satisfactory business outcomes. Because setting goals is so important, it is among the earliest decisions made.

CHOOSING A BUSINESS FORM

Another early decision is the choice of the form your business will take. The advantage of studying the various business forms before deciding which one you will adopt is that it enables you to be sure that your decision will reflect the needs and realities of your business. This saves you time and money in the long run.

As a rule, a business assumes one of three forms: (1) proprietorship, (2) partnership, or (3) corporation. There are advantages and disadvantages to each form. The purposes of the overview of business forms that follows are to acquaint you with them, to describe their commonly recognized benefits and drawbacks, and to give you material from which you can formulate questions to ask your professional advisors. You should make the actual decision about the form your business will assume only after discussing the pros and cons with your attorney, your accountant, or both. These advisors will help you determine which form best suits your specific business needs, and they are excellent sources to information on local laws and requirements in your area, as well as up-to-the-minute information on federal laws, which are currently in a state of flux.

Sole Proprietorship

Sole proprietorship, defined as a business owned and operated by one person, is the simplest form of organization. It has numerous advantages.

- It is easy to form; there are no government requirements.
- It is inexpensive to establish.
- It is easy terminate or sell the business.
- The business itself pays no taxes; all income passes to you, and you pay personal income taxes.
- Decision making is easy: you do it all.
- You are entitled to set up retirement plans for yourself.
- You maintain total control over your practice.
- You are the only person who receives any share in the profits of your company.

It also has several disadvantages.

- You have unlimited liability for the debts of your firms; that is, if you lose a suit for malpractice or negligence, or cannot pay your debts, all your assets—home, car, bank accounts, securities—will be taken to satisfy the monetary judgment against you.
- You are liable for the negligent acts of your employees.
- The business ends when you die or become disabled.
- There is less possibility of attracting venture capital.
- If the practice is sold, your profits are taxed as ordinary income (instead of at the capital gains rates, which are imposed on the sale of stock).
- You may not have all the expertise and knowledge you need to make the decisions that must be made.

Partnership

A partnership is defined as the association of two or more people to carry on a business and make a profit. There are several kinds of partnerships; the most common are the general partnership and the limited partnership. In a general partnership, the partners maintain control over the day-to-day operation of the firm. They have unlimited liability for the firm's debts, and each partner is responsible for the acts of each and every other partner. A partnership agreement between the partners specifies all aspects of the relationship. Such agreements typically cover the following points (Gray, 1985, p. 33; Riccardi & Dayani, 1982, pp. 179–180):

- the name, purpose, and location of partnership;
- the duration of the agreement;
- the names and types of partners (general, limited);
- eligibility for partnership;
- the financial contribution to be made by partners (immediate or postponed);
- the role of various partners in management of business;
- the authority of various partners in conducting the business;
- the nature and degree of each partner's contribution to the services provided by the firm;
- how business expenses will be handled;
- specification of separate debts;
- who is responsible for signing or entitled to sign checks;
- how profits and losses will be divided;
- the methods by which accounting, books, and records will be handled;
- how salaries will be drawn;
- how absence and disability will be handled;
- dissolution and winding-up upon the death of a partner;
- death benefits;
- the rights of a continuing partner;
- sale of partnership interest and retirement;

- settlement of disputes and arbitration;
- additions, alterations, or modifications to the partnership agreement;
- noncompetition in the event of departure; and
- miscellaneous (automobile, medical examinations, etc.).

In a limited partnership, the partners exert no control over day-to-day activities. These "silent partners" typically invest money or other assets into the firm and receive a share of the firm's profits or assets in return. The liability of limited partners extends only to the amount of their investment. The relationship between limited and general partners is specified in a limited partner agreement.

The advantages of a partnership are as follows.

- It is easy to form.
- Decision making is still relatively flexible.
- It is relatively free of government controls and demands.
- You can set up retirement plans for yourself and your partners.
- Venture capital is easier to attract.
- You have a greater pool of skills to draw from in running the business.
- In some respects, the business is an entity separate from the owners.

The following are the disadvantages.

- Liability is unlimited: each general partner's personal assets are subject to seizure to pay outstanding business debts.
- Individuals, not the partnership, pay taxes on business income and are responsible for for expenses.
- Partnership agreements must be rewritten when a partner dies, chooses to withdraw, or retires, or when a new partner is to be admitted.
- Control and decision-making are divided among several people.
- It may be difficult to place a value on the portion of the business that each partner owns.

Corporation

A corporation is defined as a legal entity apart from its owners; it has all the rights and responsibilities of a person, except for those rights that only a natural person can exercise. Corporations exist within the confines of charter granted by each state.

Two of the most common types of corporations are the professional corporation and the subchapter S corporation. Professional corporations provide the benefits of a corporation to people who are licensed to practice a profession. Regular corporation cannot provide services for which licensure is required. Professional corporations do not affect professional responsibility or protect those who are incorporating from liability or malpractice. Tax benefits, which have now been eliminated by the Federal Government's 1987 Budget Deficit Reduction Plan, were the major benefit realized by professionals in this type of incorporation.

Subchapter S corporations allow business owners to avoid the double taxation of corporate income and shareholder dividends and to offset business losses incurred for the corporation against their income. The regulations that govern taxation of these corporations are found in subchapter S of the Internal Revenue Code. Only corporations that are closely held (i.e., have ten or fewer shareholders initially) are eligible to make the sub-S election. Not all states recognize Sub-S incorporations.

A corporation is created when articles of incorporation are filed in the state in which the corporation will exist. The information covered by a corporation's charter typically includes (Broom, Longenecker, & Moore, 1983, p. 176)

- the name of the company;
- a formal statement of its formation;
- its purposes and powers—that is, the type of business it is;
- the location of the principal office in the state of incorporation;
- its duration (perpetual existence, 50 years, life and renewable charter, etc.);
- the classes and preferences of classes of stock;
- the number and par of stated value of shares of each class of stock authorized;
- the voting privileges of each class of stock;
- the names and addresses of incorporators and the first-year directors;

- the names and addresses of, and the amounts subscribed by, each subscriber to capital stock;
- a statement of limited liability of stockholders (required specifically by state law in many states); and
- a statement of alterations of directors' powers, if any, from the general corporation law of the state.

Once the articles of incorporation are approved, a certificate of incorporation is issued. Stockholders then transfer cash or property to the corporation and receive shares of stock in exchange. The stockholders elect a board of directors to run the corporation and officers to implement the policies the board formulates. Officers oversee the day-to-day operation of the corporation. The stockholders and the board of directors meet frequently to handle matters pertinent to the corporation.

The corporate business form has several important advantages.

- Liability is limited to the firm's assets.
- Venture capital is easier to attract than is the case with partnerships or sole proprietorships.
- There are tax advantages for pension and profit-sharing plans.
- There is a larger pool of talent for decision making.

It also has some disadvantages.

- Taxes are typically higher than for sole proprietorships or partnerships.
- It is more expensive to establish and operate a corporation.
- Government requirements can be time-consuming and cumbersome.
- The powers of the corporation are limited to those stated in the charter.
- It may be difficult to do business in another state, because of conflicting laws governing corporations.

The nurses who responded to our survey had started a total of 65 businesses; of these, 26 were sole proprietorships, nine were partnerships, and 30 were corporations. This finding tends to support the argument that no one business form is more advantageous than another except insofar as it meets specific individual needs better. The same can be said for the choices an entrepreneur makes about creating a business image.

CREATING A BUSINESS IMAGE

The image you want to project about yourself and your business is an important component of several other decisions. The "look" you develop plays a significant role in your business success, or lack thereof. It is reflected in your choice of furnishings, of cards and brochures, of business stationery, of personal presentation style, and of written communication. Before you make these choices, stop to consider how you want your clients to see you.

The nurse entrepreneurs we contacted described a variety of images they wanted to convey and linked these to the kinds of services they provided. Nurses in private practice generally wanted an environment that was warm and expressed caring and security to clients. They were also conscious of the need to be seen as competent professionals that provided a credible health-care alternative. Nurse entrepreneurs who marketed to administrators, businesses, legislators, or other nonpatient clients tended to be interested in presenting a businesslike, financially sound, and successful image. Whatever your emphasis the importance of image cannot be ignored. The following five recommendations should help you determine the most appropriate image for your business.

Understand Your Client

Make sure you ascertain what image is most likely to generate a positive response in prospective clients. Nurses establishing a private practice have a good practical understanding of patient expectations and carry that understanding into their business development; however, nurse entrepreneurs who must deal with a different type of client (businessmen, administrators, legislators, etc.) may have a more difficult time recognizing the unwritten image expectations of the "old boy" or "old girl" network in which they operate. Investigate these hidden rules ahead of time through research, observation, and your own support network.

Know Yourself

Assess your own verbal and nonverbal presentation style and compare it with client expectations. What changes, if any, do you need to make in personal skills, dress, appearance, and writing ability? You can develop a positive business image without becoming a slave to "dress for success" fads or attempting to paste a false veneer on the real you. Recognizing the message to which your clients respond and developing the skills and style that enable you to project that message effectively are essential to developing a business image.

Project Quality

Philip Holland (1984), writing about "quality without compromise," reminds entrepreneurs that "business empires are built on this single ingredient" (p. 101). This point is especially relevant to image. High quality is essential to all aspects of the enterprise, not just the service or product you provide. Whether you are selecting furnishings, business cards and brochures, letterhead stationery, or clothing, choose the best quality available. Remember that all these items say something about you and your business. Make certain that the message is consistent with the quality you want the client to associate with your service.

Use Expert Advice

Take advantage of the expertise that image experts or other entrepreneurs can provide. For example, use an artist to help you design your business card or brochure. Perhaps a marketing expert can help you develop an effective mailing, or an interior decorator who designs business office space can help you create the environment you want. Expert advice can be obtained from a variety of journals, in a university setting, from friends or family members who are experts, or from a professional with the skill you need. Nancy Doleysh hired an art student at the local university to help design the business card for Advanced Health Care Concepts, and Gerry Vogel used her husband's artistic talents to design the business card and brochure for WORKSTYLES. Remember that the experts can assist you, but it is you who must be satisfied with the end result, since the image ultimately reflects you.

Pay Attention to Detail

Since everything that represents your business says something about you, you should carefully evaluate the image you project in any type of client contact. Take the time to review written client communications for accuracy, clarity, and style. Make certain that the people who work for you share your commitment to clients and demonstrate that in their interactions with them. Many business details can be delegated to others when neceasary, but your image cannot. Paying attention to detail is essential to image making.

Image considerations also play a part in other decisions you make, such as selecting a business name or choosing an office space. For this reason, most entrepreneurs evaluate their image at an early stage of their business start-up. Once you have identified the image you want to create, you can use it as a guide to future decisions.

SELECTING A BUSINESS NAME

There are numerous factors to consider in choosing a name for a business. Basically, you can take one of two approaches to naming your business: you can use your own name, or you can create a name for the new entity. Each approach has advantages and disadvantages. If you use your own name, it may make your business sound too small; that is, it may not inspire confidence in would-be clients. On the other hand, because nurses offer a personal service and are promoting themselves, being perceived as small may actually be a drawing card for potential clients. Some nurse entrepreneurs have added "and Associates" to their name to keep the personal touch while projecting an image of extended resources.

There are other reasons why nurses choose not to use their own names. Some nurses know that they will wish to sell their business some day, and they are not comfortable with the thought that a business over which they will have no control will bear their name. Some nurses start a business in their spare time and do not wish their employer to know that they have their own business on the side. Still other nurses choose not to use their own names because they want the name to reflect their business focus.

The nurses who responded to our questionnaire were asked to answer two questions: How did you decide on the name for your business? and What special significance does the name have? The following are some representative responses.

R. Mimi Clarke Secor, of Nurse Practitioner Associates (Cambridge, MA), states,

> I decided on Nurse Practitioner Associates because I wanted to market to the world who I was, and as such, what I was up to. I didn't want any confusion as to what type of provider I was. I still have to educate clients as to what a Nurse Practitioner is, but at least they don't think I am a physician. My name was a reflection of how I wanted to be out of the closet about my identity.

Jamie Hills, of New Care Concepts, Inc., (Seattle, WA), says,

> The name was chosen to indicate that the clients we serve are treated differently than "traditional" home health agencies. My idea for a new care concept was to provide stable, long-term staffing, eliminating the revolving door syndrome and providing medical and dental insurance and job stability for the nursing staff.

Sheila Quilter Wheeler, of Wheeler and Associates (San Anselmo, CA) remarks,

> The name I'm using is temporary—I have vacillated between several others, and this seems to sum up with the image I want to project—no-

nonsense, businesslike, even if it doesn't tell exactly what we do. My other possible choice is Telephone Triage Associates; for some reason, I find this limiting.

Carolyn Edison, of Family Health Care, Inc. (Liberty, MO), explains her name simply:

Family—oriented toward the entire family; Health—synonymous with nursing; Care—consistent with our philosophy of nursing.

Barbara Klein, from Capistrano Beach, CA, uses her own name because she feels it has more credibility than a constructed/created name.

Judy Dean, of Health Care Consultants of Wisconsin (Sussex, WI), explains,

We went through many possible names, some catchy, and finally determined that the name had to convey what we did. We did not include "education" in the name, as we wanted the option at a future date to expand our services. We felt that the name conveyed our ability to consult in health-care concerns in any arena that we chose to pursue.

Marcia Harris, of Home Hospice Nursing, Inc. (LaGrange, IL), remarks,

The name is short, simple, to the point, and highly descriptive of services. Other names for this type of business were either too religious, too cutesy, or too maudlin.

Carole Meola, of Management and Career Resources (Norfolk, VA), explains her choice vividly:

Tell it like it is! Management and Career Resources—we are an organization that deals in information and resources.

Nancy Dirubbo, of Laconia Women's Health Center (Laconia, NH), notes,

I wanted to identify the location, target population, and not limit the name to pure medical nursing care. This will allow me to add other health disciplines as growth occurs. I am the only women's health center in a 45-mile radius.

Penny Hamlin and Jane Aral, of Nurse Edu-Care/Resource Network (NEC/RN) (Alliance, OH), say,

We brainstormed on the name, came up with the idea that we wanted the name to reflect *what* we did and to have a catchy, shorter name. We are a resource educational network of caring nurses: NEC/RN (the NEC can imply that we are necessary RNs)."

Dr. Barbara Bohny, of New Hope Respite and Home Care (Haledon, NJ), states,

> New Hope implies hope for families caring for a loved one at home.

Donna Ipema, of Associates in Counseling (Oak Park, IL), explains,

> We chose a name that started with A, as that would be first in a Yellow Pages. "Counseling" was accurate and seemed acceptable to the public.

Lorraine Jacobson, of Wingspan (Marysville, WA), notes that

> Wingspan is a concept of what I do: helping people go from position A (where they are) to position B (where they want to be) with the ease of an eagle's wing.

Joell Archibald, of The Warming Touch (Tacoma, WA), observes,

> Many, many, many hours were spent brainstorming with other business professionals in my MBA coursework and with nursing peers. I felt that the business name needed to be representative of the special contribution nurses make while exercising their skills, that it needed to be descriptive of the service I planned to offer, and that it be broad enough to retain once the level of services offered was expanded.

(Warming Touch provides assessment of the jaundiced infant, parent instruction and teaching on newborn issues, blood work, and provision of phototherapy when ordered by the physician, all done in the family's home.)

Mary Ellen Stone of Stone and Associates (Stanhope, NY), states,

> I researched consulting and decided that the name should avoid a cute or clever appearance. Instead, it should sound long-standing; hence, Stone and Associates.

Elizabeth Dayani of American Nursing Resources (Overland, KS) is simply observes that "American starts with an A for Yellow Pages listing."

Michael Johnson, of Consulting Opinion, Inc. (Seattle, WA), explains,

> I felt clients sought *consulting* services as a means of obtaining a neutral, objective *opinion*—thus the name.

Karen Hyland, of Professional Resources in Nursing, Inc. (Kansas City, MO), states,

> The name of the firm was intended to imply that this corporation could provide more than one specialty in nursing resources. The name allows for continued expansion of nursing services as demands for additional specialties continue. The name can be shortened to PRN—advertisting appeal.

Susan Reuler of Professional Nursing Associates (Denver, CO), explains,

> The name was decided on over a dinner with my father. We felt that our nurses needed to feel ownership—i.e., "Associates"—"Professional" for the association, and "Nursing" to identify our target market.

Susan Donaldson of Independent Nursing Services (Oil City, PA), states,

> We wanted to convey the fact that we were operating on an "independent" basis and were not affiliated with any hospitals or agencies. We chose a name which would reflect what we were readily, so there would be no guesswork for the potential client.

Dolores Alford, of the Institute of Gerontic Nursing (Dallas, TX), notes,

> Institute was chosen for its academic/research connotation. Gerontic refers to all facets of aging—and, of course, we wanted nursing identification. The name is significant because it demonstrates the emerging sophistication of nursing in a specialty of great importance.

The thought processes used in selecting an appropriate business name varied greatly among the nurse entrepreneurs who responded to the questionnaire. You may find it helpful to consider how they chose their names as you decide what you want your name to say about your business.

LOCATING A SPACE FOR THE BUSINESS

Selecting office space is as crucial as choosing a business name. The decision about where to work affects time management, the image you present to clients, and your own sense of well-being as a businessperson. Your selection will depend on a variety of factors, the most important of which are expense, convenience, appeal to clients, and the special needs of the business. Each of the two options, a home office and a office space outside the home, has benefits and drawbacks.

The Home Office

Like many of the nurse entrepreneurs whose experience we drew on for this book, both of us chose to have our office in our homes. Several benefits made this an obvious choice. First, there are the financial benefits: no overhead for office space and the ability to use the home office as a business tax deduction. Second, a home office allows considerable personal flexibility, which is vital when an entrepreneur is balancing numerous responsibilities. You are available for family needs, should they arise, and you can more easily pick up your work at odd hours (e.g., 2 AM) when those other needs have been met if your office is only a few steps away. Third, you can exercise personal choice in the design of the office space when it is part of your own home.

The home office also has disadvantages. The most significant of these is that it is difficult to protect your work time from others, as well as from yourself. Family, friends, and community groups (like the PTA) frequently presume that you are available whenever you are at home, and it is hard to separate personal tasks from business tasks when you work at home. After all, why not vacuum the living room before starting that project report? There are several "time wasters" lurking in your home; consequently, good time management tactics are essential. Mary Ellen Stone, of Stone and Associates, provides health, critical care, and management education, as well as consulting services, to a variety of businesses and health-care organizations from her home office. She makes use of three strategies to stay in control of her business time.

> I go straight to my office in the AM with coffee. I make all calls initially in the morning, as this frees me to complete tasks later. Once or twice a week, I arrange to see an appointment outside the home.

As Mary Ellen Stone has discovered, good time management skills are a must when you work at home.

Another possible disadvantage to a home office is that it does not present a positive business image to potential clients; for this reason, the home office works best when the entrepreneur goes to see clients rather than the reverse. This disadvantage can, however, be eliminated through planning, if you select and remodel a home space in such a way to give you both privacy and a good business image.

If you choose to have your office in your home, the following suggestions can help you to create an optimal working environment.

1. Develop separate work and personal time schedules, and stick to them.
2. Limit personal interruptions to your business time. This may involve assertive negotiation and planning with family members, using an answering machine to block unnecessary phone messages, or just learning to say no.

3. Select and organize a specific space that is used as your work space and nothing else. Unless you do this, your home office expenses are not fully tax-deductible. In addition, it is too difficult to move work materials from the dining room table every evening. Furthermore, this "nomad office" syndrome does not contribute to your business self-concept or to your image as an entrepreneur.
4. Create the kind of esthetic environment that is important for you—plants, art work, etc. This will make moving into your work mode that much easier.
5. Invest in office furniture that will allow you to collect and organize the necessary equipment, supplies, and files in the most efficient way.
6. If you will be seeing clients in your home, remember to consider the image you want to present as you make decisions about suggestions 4 and 5.
7. Remember to check the zoning regulations for home offices in your locality, as well as any changes in liability coverage that affect home offices.

The Traditional Office Solution

The home office is a convenient alternative, but it is not right for everyone. Many nurses prefer an outside business office, for several important reasons. A traditional office can appear more businesslike to clients, and its location may communicate an important message. Linda Hackett and Lenore Boles, of Nurse Counseling Group, had a specific point in mind when they chose their office site.

> We have offices on "doctor's row" in Norwalk. From the beginning we decided to openly compete with the physicians and give the message that we give high-quality professional care.

Image questions aside, the traditional office is less vulnerable to intrusion from nonbusiness sources than the home office is. When Sheila Quilter Wheeler started Wheeler and Associates, a consulting service for the design, training, and implementation of Telephone Triage Systems, she worked in her home. Within a year, she moved to an office outside her home.

> I now share a small office with another consultant in an older office building close to where I live. It is a much more satisfactory situation than sharing my office with a washer and a dryer and two kids pounding on the door.

Other reasons for choosing a traditional office are a need for space, because of the number of employees to be hired or the amount or size of the equipment needed for the business; client convenience; ease of client access to the site; and increased visibility in the client market. Whatever the reason for the choice, there are several factors to consider in selecting a site:

1. Is the space adequate for current needs and for possible expansion?
2. Can clients easily gain access to the building? Is there adequate parking?
3. Is the location convenient for you?
4. What image do the location and the building itself project?
5. What are the overhead costs? How frequently have they increased in the past?
6. Does the office design (light, windows, view, etc.) meet your own esthetic requirements?

The major disadvantages associated with traditional office space are rising costs; failure to maintain the condition of the building; problems with other tenants in the building; and gradual loss of businesses from the area, leaving your office isolated and decreasing its value as a place of business. Taking the time to investigate the present site for suitability now and in the future is one way of avoiding some of these problems. Making certain that you have an explicit contract with options to terminate a lease clearly identified is another. Sharing or subletting office space can help to defray part of the cost.

Once you have an office, you must determine which support services are necessary to operate that office. You may decide to hire a secretary or purchase a computer, or you may opt to purchase services on a need basis. At this point, you should try to identify the types of support or equipment services you will need.

SUPPORT AND EQUIPMENT SERVICES

Decisions about support and equipment services are important, since they dramatically affect start-up costs. For example, it may be more cost-effective to purchase computer services than to invest in a $3,000 to $5,000 system at start-up. Thus, you may choose to rent certain support services on an as-needed basis rather than hire someone or purchase the equipment necessary. Knowing the cost of each option will help you make a better-informed decision. Recently, the development of identity plans and incubator organizations has presented the entrepreneur with two unique ways of acquiring support services.

The Identity Plan

An identity plan is designed to address the support problems that new business owners and small business owners face. Frequently, entrepreneurs' requirements for space or for a specific type of service, such as a secretary, vary considerably from month to month or even week to week. These services can be provided on an as-needed basis, which saves entrepreneurs the full-time expense of the services or specialized space. Alice Marie Kotkowski, of AMK Associates, uses this method to acquire the support services that are not available in her home-based office.

> Only in incidents of recruiting do clients come to me. I always go to them. So I work out of a formal home office, but utilize an identity plan that provides a mailing address, telephone services, secretarial and computer services, and hourly cost rental of a conference or boardroom when needed. This is a new service (three years old) that is spreading nationally.

Identity plans give you the best of both worlds: a home office and a traditional office environment.

The Incubator Organization

Incubator organizations allow new entrepreneurs to acquire office space and a variety of centralized services at relatively low cost, including secretarial, billing, and computer services. The costs of these services is shared by each business. The entrepreneur can often purchase specialized assistance, such as market testing and business plan development. Because many incubators demand a percentage of the business from entrepreneurs who join, this option must be weighed carefully.

Either of these two options can extend the buying power of the new entrepreneur. You can check on the availability of identity plans or incubators in the business section of your local newspaper; in the local business newspaper or journal, if one is published in your community; or with the Small Business Association. Since decisions about support and equipment services will influence your start-up costs, this is a good time to evaluate your needs and balance them with the cost and availability of various options. Exercise 5.1 lists some common support services and equipment that entrepreneurs use. Determine whether your needs for a particular service are continuous or episodic; ascertain the cost and availability of different ways of obtaining that service; and complete the exercise.

✔ **Exercise 5.1 Typical Support Services and Equipment for a Business.**

Instructions. Place a check in the "Yes" or the "No" column to indicate whether you need each of these services. Place checks in the other columns to indicate how you plan to acquire these services.

Service Equipment	Need: Yes	Need: No	Hire or Buy	Rent as Needed	Cost
Secretary					
Computer					
Mailing					
Printing					
Copying					
Payroll					
Cleaning					
Accounting					
Audiovisual					
Other (list)					

You will use the results of this exercise in chapter 7 to determine part of your start-up costs. Decisions about purchased services should be made before decisions about supplies and equipment, since you may not need certain equipment, such as a computer, if you elect to rent the related service.

SELECTING OFFICE SUPPLIES AND EQUIPMENT

Although each business will create a demand for different kinds and amounts of supplies and equipment, there are certain basic needs for every office. To help you collect all the appropriate accessories and to estimate probable costs, we have complied a checklist of essential, optional, and specialty items. The cost of these items will very, depending on the amount purchased, the quality (in some instances), and the locale in which they were purchased. Take this checklist along to office equipment and supply stores and note prices for items you know you need. Then do some comparative shopping for the bit items, so that you are not thrown into a state of cardiac arrest the first time you walk out with a $300.00 bill for "basic supplies."

✔ Exercise 5.2 Office Start-Up Checklist.

Instructions. Place a check in the "Need" column after each of the items you need, and make a note of the appropriate quantity. Then, when you have determined the price you will pay for each item, enter that in the appropriate space.

Item	Needed	Quantity	Cost
Basic Supplies			
Pens			
Erasers			
Pencils			
Whiteout			
Paperclips			
Lined paper			
Legal-size pads			
Typing paper			
Files			
Desk pad			
Manila folders			
Envelopes			
Staples			
Paper cutter			
Three-hole punch			
Ruler			
Pencil sharpener			
Scotch tape			
Scissors			
Pocket calendar			
Memo pads			
Equipment			
Typewriter			
Word processor			
Computer			
Telephone			
Answering machine			
Beeper			
Copier			

Item	Needed	Quantity	Cost
Calculator			
Office furniture			
Desk			
Typing table			
Computer station			
Bookcases			
Files			
Lamps			
Chairs			
Drapes			
Carpeting			
Artwork			
Clinical practice equipment			
(list)			
Business logo paper supplies			
Business cards			
Brochures			
Letterhead paper			
Letterhead envelopes			
Statements			
Audio visual equipment			
Flip chart and pad			
Transparencies			
Transparency markers			
Tape recorder			
Slide projector			
Movie projector			
video recorder			
Slide camera			

This list is intended to give an idea of what goes into a new business office and to help you estimate your start-up costs. Having the supplies and equipment you need will promote an efficient environment; still, however, the most significant influence on organizational effectiveness is a well-defined work process.

ESTABLISHING A WORK PROCESS

Peter Drucker (1987) makes a useful distinction between efficiency and effectiveness: "Efficiency is getting everything done right. Effectiveness is getting the right things done" (p. 2). Establishing a work process that is both efficient and effective is vital for start-up undertaking. It includes six steps:

1. identifying the priority activities of the business day,
2. integrating time management practices,
3. developing a communication process,
4. developing employee teams,
5. evaluating outcomes on a continuing basis, and
6. personal and professional development.

Priority Activities

Ensuring that the "right things" get done necessitates conscious decisions about the priority activities of each day. Your goals should govern these decisions: if a particular activity is not helping you meet your goals, eliminate it or delegate it. For example, in a clinical practice, the quality of the time you spend with patients may be the single most important work consideration, influencing how you structure your work patterns or respond to interruptions during that time. If this is in fact a priority, perhaps you should not be doing your own typing, billing, or other office work. Deciding now what your priority business activities are will guide you in structuring a satisfying work process and help you to realize when you are not using time profitably and should eliminate or arrange for help with inappropriate activities.

Time Management

Integrate time management strategies early. Ask yourself what time blocks you are most likely to experience. Then, from the very first day, take steps to avoid these blocks. Set limits on interruptions, learn to say "no", and divide large projects into their component parts so that you can complete pieces of that task within relatively short periods. If it helps, make a "to do" list. Most important, make sure that *you* make the decisions about your time. After all, independence is probably one of the reasons why you became an entrepreneur.

Communication Process

Establish mechanisms for sharing and receiving information. When and how do you contact clients? How do you keep employees and colleagues informed? Have you allocated the time necessary to influence others who play a part in determining whether or not your "right things" get done? To establish a pattern for business communication that will allow you to handle the information flow skillfully, ask yourself, Whom must I contact? What needs to be communicated? How will I communicate? and When (how frequently) will I communicate?

Developing Work Teams

If you have employees, partners, or associates, it's important that you begin a planned team building process that will result in the formation of a motivated, cohesive work group made up of people who support each other and the goals of the business. Make sure that roles are clearly defined and that the dimensions of individual power and accountability are recognized and supported within the team. When conflicts occur, encourage open, honest communication, and help with the development of feedback skills when necessary. Unresolved conflicts hinder individual and organizational attainment of goals and are frequently a signal that team-building efforts are long overdue.

Evaluate Outcomes

Maintain an in-depth knowledge of what is happening in your business. Continual assessment of results achieved; failed initiatives; expenditure of time, money, and energy; and income generated is essential for monitoring the vitality of the business. Success often depends on such vigilance.

Developing Personally and Professionally

Clients request your services because of your professional skills. This creates an ongoing need for growth and change, which makes professional development a priority activity. Plans for meeting this need should therefore be considered when you start your business. In addition, the challenges of running a business place additional demands and new stresses on you. As you plan your work process, remember to include opportunities for developing personal strengths, insights, and new coping strategies. Entrepreneurial burnout is not a business goal.

The reason why it is important to consider these six steps at this stage of the business endeavor is that it is much easier to institute an effective work process initially than to attempt to undo a dysfunctional process later on in response to a chaotic situation. Taking the time now to analyze your needs and institute a functional process will make a well-organized business start-up easier to achieve.

DEVELOPING AN ORGANIZED DOCUMENTATION PROCESS

Documents that organize daily business operations also facilitate the smooth flow of business activity. Requirements for particular organizing documents vary considerably, depending on the specific type of business you have developed.

Nurses in Private Practice

Nurses who provide direct patient care are faced with a wide range of prescribed documents that are necessary for reimbursement. Medicare/Medicaid and other third-party insurer forms, for example, demand a great deal of paperwork and considerable attention to detail. In addition to these prescribed forms, the nurse in private practice must generate other documents for internal organiziation purposes, such as clinical records, nurse's notes, patient education materials, or patient authorization forms for release of information. If you are starting a clinical practice, you should consult nurse entrepreneurs with similar practices or a lawyer familiar with practice-model businesses to determine what the essential documents are for you.

The Nurse Employer

If you are an employer, personnel documentation creates an additional paper network. Necessary forms include personnel policies and procedures, job descriptions, evaluation tools, payroll records, time cards, evidence of licensure, tax withholding records, employee health forms, and work schedules. Given the complexity of the federal and labor regulations that govern recordkeeping, expert advice about personnel documentation is advisable and should be sought from your attorney or accountant.

The Nurse Consultant

Nurse consultants require special documents in order to organize the practice, develop proposals for potential clients, legitimize agreements with clients, establish mutually agreed-upon objectives for the consulting interaction, set fees, and prevent unnecessary legal problems. The documents that the consultant most often needs to create are a proposal format, a client contract, and subcontracting agreements. Each of these is discussed more fully in chapter 9; samples of these documents are included in Appendix 4.

Since a nurse entrepreneur may function in a variety of roles, his or her documentation needs may fall into several of the categories discussed. Use the checklist provided in Exercise 5.3 to identify the documentation needs of your business.

✔ Exercise 5.3 Document Checklist.

Instructions. Place a check next to the documents that you need in your business.

Private practice
Insurance forms (list) ________

Clinical records ________
Nurse's notes ________
Progress notes ________
Patient education record ________
Information release ________
Medication record ________
Nursing assessment ________
Patient education materials ________
Appointment cards

Employer
Application forms ________
Employment interview forms ________
Job descriptions ________
Performance evaluation ________
Policies and procedures ________
Employment termination ________
Payroll records ________
Time card ________
Tax witholding ________
Employee health forms ________
Schedule of hours ________

Employer (cont.)
Evidence of licensure ________
Grievance procedure ________
Employment contract ________
Employee handbook ________

Consulting
Proposals ________
Contracts ________
Subcontract agreements ________

All businesses
Purchase orders ________
Billing statements ________

This list is not meant to be all inclusive; it is intended merely to remind you of your documentation needs. Documents, if properly selected, can help to increase overall order and efficiency. Unnecessary documentation, however, is to be avoided at all costs: If a document does not add to the organizing efforts of the business, change it or get rid of it.

A FINAL LOOK AT ORGANIZING

We have presented a variety of details that you should consider in developing a systematic process for handling the daily activities of a new business and have illustrated these with examples of how other entrepreneurs have organized their start-up period. We recognize that your business is unique, and you will discover creative ways to organize; we have provided this information in an effort to save you from having to reinvent the wheel. In Exercise 5.4, use the material presented to begin making organizing decisions. The choices made at this time will influence your business costs, your feelings of control, and your marketing efforts in the future.

✔ Exercise 5.4 **Organizing Decisions.**

Instructions. Complete each of the following statements.

1. My business philosophy is:

2. My business goals (if they have changed since I listed them in chapter 3) are:

3. The ideal form for my business is:

   My reasons for choosing this form are:

4. The image I want to project is:

5. The name I have chosen for my business is:

6. My ideal office location is:

7. The priority activities that I want to spend time on daily are:

8. The time traps I am most likely to encounter are:

   My strategies for improving my time management are:

9. My daily communication priorities include (the who, what, when, and how of information processing):

10. I assess how the business is doing as follows:

What Is To Be Evaluated	How	When

11. My personal development plan is:

    My professional development plan is:

12. I need the following documentation to do business:

Necessary Documents	Need to Develop	Need to Obtain

By this point, you have considered the major questions about how to organize a business start-up. Your ability to answer the questions in Exercise 5.4 is an indicator of whether you need to carry out further research to make an informed decision. When you can ask the right questions and know where to locate the sources of information, you are in business.

6 MARKETING A NURSING BUSINESS

Most nurses have limited experience with marketing, because the responsibility for marketing is traditionally assumed by the agencies that employ them. This inexperience increases a nurse entrepreneur's susceptibility to three major marketing mistakes:

1. not realizing that marketing is important,
2. failing to develop a marketing plan, and
3. using inappropriate marketing strategies.

To avoid these mistakes, you must acquire an understanding of basic marketing concepts and their special application to nurse-run businesses, a knowledge of effective promotion strategies, and the ability to develop a marketing plan.

BASIC MARKETING CONCEPTS

The basic marketing concepts that we will be discussing here are the definition of marketing, the relevance of marketing to business outcomes, and the relationship of the five critical marketing components to a nurse-run business.

Definition of Marketing

According to Levinson (1984, p.3),

> Marketing is everything you do to promote your business from the moment you conceive of it to the point at which customers buy your product or service and begin to patronize your business on a regular basis. The key words to remember are *everything* and *regular basis*.

This definition illustrates the pervasive influence marketing has on all aspects of business operations. The marketing process illustrated in Figure 6.1 is

	I Assessment	II Analysis	III Planning	IV Action	V Evaluation
	The Company				
Internal	Goals Resources Culture Current Market Quality Assurance	Status of Internal Environment	Target Markets	Operationalize Plan	Evaluate Outcomes
	Trend Analysis	Emerging Trends	Identify Organizational Changes		
	Expectations-Values Knowledge/Technology Demographic Regulatory Professional	Emerging Markets	Develop Plan Goals Objectives Personnel Resources Time Table		
External	Market Research	Status of Current Market			
	New Clients Competition Public Image				

Figure 6.1 Components of the Marketing Process.

integral to routine planning, evaluation, and decisions about expenditure of resources (time, money, and energy). The assessment phase generates information through market research and trend analysis (see chapter 3) as well as an evaluation of the business itself. These data are analyzed in the second stage with the aim of predicting potential markets, identifying the status of current markets, and determining the organization's marketing capabilities for handling current and future client demands. Next, a plan is developed that targets markets and mobilizes organizational capacity to meet demands. Finally, the plan is operationalized and its outcomes evaluated. The process is continuous and drives the operation efforts of the business. The relevance of the marketing process to successful business development is the reason for its importance as an organizational function.

Relevance of Marketing

A planned marketing process offers four benefits to businesses: (1) it generates clients, (2) it provides trend analysis for growth decisions, (3) it assesses the competition, and (4) it assists with pricing decisions. Each of these benefits contributes to determining the success of the start-up and growth phases of the enterprise.

Generating Clients. It is not enough simply to offer a quality service: you must also convince clients to use that service. Market research targets clients who need your service, specifies the strategies that will influence clients to use your service rather those of your competitor's, and alerts you to prospective clients on a continuing basis.

Trend Analysis. The main value of trend analysis is that it discourages complacency, preventing you from being lulled by success. Success is of course your goal, but it can be dangerous when it "encourages the viewpoint that the future is a mirror of the past" (Hartley, 1986, p.287). Trend analysis is closely linked to business survival because it presents the entrepreneur with significant clues to new opportunities and predicts potential changes in the need for services currently in demand. It is a future-oriented strategy.

Assessing the Competition. In addition to identifying prospective clients, market research evaluates the status of a business relative to its competition. Specifically, it tells you how your market share compares to that of the competition and how your business measures up to the competition in terms of quality, new services or products offered, and pricing structure. This information helps you to locate the aspects of your service that are unique, as well as offers clues to marketing strategies for maintaining or increasing your client base.

Pricing Structure. As the market for, demand for, and availability of specific services change, the prices charged for those services also begin to fluctuate. Paying attention to any alterations in the diverse variables that influence the market value of your services puts you in a position to formulate pricing strategies that ensure a profit without discouraging potential clients.

Making a commitment to marketing as a vital part of operating a business is the first step toward effective marketing. Learning to manage the controllable marketing variables to your advantage is the second.

Five Essential Components of a Marketing Program

There are five variables that an entrepreneur can control or direct in order to market a service or product: (1) the firm's public image (its reputation, how it and its outputs are perceived); (2) the nature, quality, and features of the product; (3) the price to be charged for the product; (4) the promotion of the product; and (5) the distribution or placement of the product in the market (Hartley, 1984). Public image has a direct impact on each of the other four variables, and all five variables have a bearing on the difficulties experienced in marketing a nurse run business.

Nurses face certain marketing challenges common to most other persons who offer professional services to clients. (Bloom, 1984):

1. clients' lack of understanding about nurses and nursing services;
2. the difficulty of explaining to clients the significant differences between nurse providers and other health-care providers, or between different nurse providers;
3. clients' inability to assess experience and competence in nurse providers; and
4. the traditional lack of direct reimbursement for nursing services, which fosters an unwillingness to pay nurses at a level with similarly prepared providers in other professions.

To address these marketing problems effectively, nurse entrepreneurs must be proficient at managing the five marketing variables listed above. Understanding how each of these variables affects the marketing of a nursing business makes it possible to use them strategically.

Public Image. Nurse entrepreneurs must contend with the images that their various publics have of them. These images may be positive, negative, or neutral; in fact, different publics may have several different images of the same nurse. Your image can have a considerable effect on your business; consequently, you must take pains to evaluate exactly how you are perceived by the groups with whom you interact.

Positive images—perceptions of you as competent, independent, businesslike, or the provider of a valued service—will allow you to generate and keep clients more readily. If you have a positive image, it is important to recognize it and to use it as a marketing asset. Ruth Halverson, a nurse midwife who owns Ruth's Maternity/GYN clinic, used a positive image to her advantage in two ways.

> I took over an established practice, The Mount Vernon Birth Center, in 1979, so I didn't have to do a lot of marketing. Since I have worked in this area for 12 years, I have been known as "Ruth." That is why I chose to change the business name and use mine.

The point of this example is that a positive image may be of little or no use to you if you do not realize that you have it, recognize its source, and understand how to capitalize on it in your marketing efforts.

Negative images—perceptions of you as dependent, victimized, insufficiently knowledgeable, or too costly—are difficult to overcome. Usually, they must be counteracted by a strong marketing program. Among the strategies that are helpful are

1. documentation of positive image points—for example, statistics demonstrating that nursing care to patients in the home costs less than in-patient care;
2. references from previous clients;
3. a demonstration project with desired results clearly identified and tied into a contract for services; and
4. networking within the groups that represent your various publics, for the specific purpose of changing your poor image.

Neutral images present problems because they indicate a lack of awareness of nurses' capabilities and competencies. If your potential clients are undecided about or hostile to a particular image, they will be unwilling to consider using the service or reluctant to pay a price that is appropriate to the quality of the service provided.

If your publics have widely differing images of you and your services, you must make an effort to resolve the discrepancies to prevent potentially damaging conflict. For example, a patient may have a positive image of you as a competent caregiver providing a needed service, but the third-party payer may see you as poorly prepared to understand the financial side of health care or as providing an unnecessary service. In this situation, you should act to reinforce the patient's image and modify the third-party payer's image.

Because public image is so important to the nurse entrepreneur, your efforts to maintain, enhance, or develop your image must be virtually increasing. The following four guidelines should prove useful.

1. Remember that image cannot be taken for granted, and continually assess how you are perceived by your publics.
2. Evaluate the varied images your publics have of you, and market yourself to each public group appropriately.
3. Use marketing strategies that increase public understanding of who you are and what you do. For example, Nancy Dirubbo of Laconia Women's Health Center, "joined the Chamber of Commerce, donated a wellness evaluation to the local public TV auction, and contracted to have a brochure with the welcome wagon" to increase public awareness and understanding of her services.
4. Remember that your ability to favorably control the other four marketing variables depends on your ability to project a positive image.

Product. In nurse-run businesses, the product is usually a service, and the public's view of the value and quality of that service is tied to its perceptions of nurses and nursing. Frequently, the public is as perplexed about how to evaluate the service provided as it is about how to define nursing. In addition, objective measures of the quality of a service are difficult to explain, except in terms of a client's problems. For you, as a nurse entrepreneur, this means that marketing a service successfully will depend on increasing prospective clients' appreciation of your expertise and competence as a provider, as well as on demonstrating the unique ways in which your service helps clients meet pressing needs. Whether the special need is cost, availability, relief from pain or suffering, or help in developing coping skills or managerial excellence, clients must be convinced that you alone can offer solutions that meet their needs. Client education and quality assurance are both essential marketing strategies for gaining acceptance for a nursing service. Product acceptance and public image both influence pricing strategy.

Pricing. Your pricing decisions reflect your assessment of how your service is perceived by clients. If your image is that of a high-quality provider who offers a unique and highly valued service, charge a prestige price for that service. To do otherwise might put off those clients who associate price with quality. Alice-Marie Kotkowski, of AMK Associates, discovered how pricing strategy influences clients' perceptions.

> A Fortune 200 company offered a substantial piece of business with a request for an additional fee discount, giving me 24 hours to reply. I stuck to my fee because (1) my services are worth it and (2) how could I return to the old fee for smaller assignments? The corporate decision: they accepted with the statement, "you have a high price for a high-quality service." The manager's attitude showed they respected me for not selling cheap and respecting myself.

If you feel that you do not yet meet the criteria for prestige pricing, you have three other options.

First, you may choose to meet the market price of the competition. Find out what entrepreneurs with similar backgrounds and services are charging, and set your fees accordingly. Remember to keep an eye on the competition and raise your prices as theirs change. As you develop expertise or establish a feature or features unique to your services, consider raising your fees.

Second, you may charge the same fees as the competition but use a sliding scale approach to introduce new services or to encourage large-volume contracts. The danger of this strategy is that you may wind up working harder than the competition but earning less.

Third, you may charge a lower fee than the competition. Low prices may attract a flock of new clients, but there are two risks you must take into account: (1) you may, again, be overworked and underpaid, and (2) some clients may believe that low prices necessarily indicate low-quality service.

Inexperience with fee-for-service interactions predisposes nurses to underprice their services. It also makes them uncomfortable with negotiating a price or standing firm once they set a reasonable fee. If pricing is difficult for you initially, find a mentor or hire a financial advisor to help you develop a pricing strategy. Once your pricing policy is set, you can determine your promotion and placement strategies.

Promotion and Placement. The term *promotion* refers to the marketing strategies you use to sell your services to clients; *placement* refers to the strategies you use to distribute your service in client markets. These two variables are closely linked with each other and with the other three marketing variables as well. For example, if you are marketing your business as an innovative, prestigious, highly desirable service, then your price must refect this, your public image must be strong, your product/service must be of high quality, and your promotional efforts must be focused on the prestige image you desire.

Possible placement decisions include being the innovator or the first one to provide the service; offering a service provided by others, but adding a unique feature that differentiates you from the competition; being the most cost-effective provider; delivering unusually high quality; or targeting a special segment of the population.

Decisions about promotion are based on your evaluation of your public image, the demand for your services, and the desired placement of the business. These influence both your marketing goals and the strategies you must adopt to meet them. An effective promotion program has four possible goals, which evolve from the assessment described above:

1. to promote clients' awareness of the service;
2. to promote clients' understanding of the service;

3. to develop clients' perception of a need for the service; and
4. to develop clients' commitment to using the service.

Once established, these goals determine which specific promotional activities are appropriate.

PROMOTION STRATEGIES

Table 6.1 illustrates the relationship between frequently used promotion strategies and specific marketing goals. A good marketing program will contain a mix of strategies and allow you to alter that mix as your market assessment changes. You are not limited to the choices described here; most entrepreneurs develop additional creative marketing approaches. What is critical is that selection of strategies should be based on thorough analysis and planning.

For anyone planning a marketing program—especially those doing so for the first time—it may be useful to know what works for other entrepreneurs in similar businesses. Table 6.2 compares the success rates of the various promotional strategies used by nurse entrepreneurs who contributed to this book.

The most commonly used strategies have a variety of advantages and disadvantages, and their potential results must be weighed carefully against their cost.

Personal Contact

A review of Tables 6.1 and 6.2 makes it clear that personal contact is a highly successful strategy and that it is useful for meeting all four of the goals mentioned earlier. Successful personal promotion of a service, however, is the result of planning and preparation. As Connor and Davidson (1985) note,

> Effective personal selling requires that you have or develop the willingness and ability to sense the unmet needs of key clients and prospects, probe for needed information without upsetting the contact, and listen to and understand the contacts' needs and expectations. It also means that you communicate persuasively in language the client understands and, when appropriate, obtain commitment to proceed to a logical next step in the business development process.

Nurses have many of the skills mentioned or implied in this description. These skills can readily be transferred to personal contact situations if four simple guidelines are kept in mind.

TABLE 6.1 Relationships Between Strategies and Marketing Goals

Strategies	Goals			
	Client Awareness	Client Understanding	Create Client-Perceived Need	Client Contracts
Advertising	X	X	X	
Business cards	X			
Brochures	X	X	X	
Personal contact	X	X	X	X
Lectures	X	X	X	
Mailings	X	X		
Workshops/seminars	X	X	X	
Publishing	X	X	X	
Press releases	X			
Information interviews	X	X		
Hospitality suites	X	X		
Telephone contact	X	X	X	
Professional organizations	X	X		
Limited trials or demonstrations	X	X	X	X

TABLE 6.2 Success Rates of Selected Marketing Strategies Employed by 63 Nurse Entrepreneurs

	Success Rate (Number of Nurse Entrepreneurs)					
		Poor	Fair	Excellent		
Strategies	1	2	3	4	5	6
Advertising						
Newspaper	5	4	5	10	1	3
Professional journals	6	5	5	4	1	
Radio	6	2	5			2
TV	5			2	1	
Other (please list)						
Personal contact			2	4	21	36
Mailings	4	1	13	13	7	4
Telephone contact		1	11	15	9	11
Providing lectures		4	14	12	14	11
Hospitality suites	5	1	1			
Publishing	1	1	5	3	3	3
Workshops, seminars		1	7	8	14	12
Listing in telephone books	6	12	11	9	5	7
Referrals from previous clients			1	4	9	40
Referrals from other health-care providers	2		2	7	13	28

Other
- Cards and brochures
- Booth at health fairs
- Referrals from corporations
- Activity in professional organizations
- Business digest listings
- Trade shows
- Association directories
- Vendors
- Participation in community organizations
- Obtaining feedback from clients to determine satisfaction and emerging needs

1. Begin your interaction with a discussion of the client's perceived needs and problems.
2. Capture the client's attention early with needs-related statements—for example: "The latest survey indicated that 40 percent of all critical care staff nursing positions remain vacant. What impact does this figure have on staffing efficiency, productivity, and the morale of remaining staff?"
3. Describe your services in client-centered terms, that is, what outcomes the client will achieve through your services.
4. Close the interaction with a commitment to use your services. "Let's set goals and target dates so you can see progress as soon as possible."

An extension of the personal contact approach is a limited trial that provides a client with selected aspects of a service over a specific period. This option allows you to demonstrate precisely how your interventions will meet the client's needs.

Two other person-to-person approaches are the information interview and telephone contact. In the information interview, you simply explain your services and perhaps leave written information with that client. Since you are not selling at this time, the client is more likely to listen openly and remember you when future needs arise. This strategy also serves as a networking device for increasing the number of persons aware of the services you provide. Follow these four guidelines during each information interview.

1. Let the client know that your purpose is information sharing, not selling.
2. Honor that "information only" commitment during the interview.
3. Be concise: stick to any time limit established.
4. Leave written material explaining your client-centered services with the person. In fact, leave extra copies, because these can be given to other potential clients.

Telephone contact increases client awareness, but the lack of face-to-face interaction limits its effectiveness. It can, however, help to locate pockets of interest that can be followed up with personal contact.

Referrals

Referrals from previous clients are also among the most positive promotional strategies, followed closely by referrals from other health professionals. Word-of-mouth referrals often happen serendipitously; however, any strategy that generates such good results should be made part of a planned marketing effort. Can you include recommendations from clients or other health care professionals as part of your other strategies (e.g. brochures or advertising)?

Hospitality Suites

Hosting a hospitality suite during a convention increases your visibility to a broad base of clients and gives you an opportunity to explain your services and distribute cards and brochures. This is an expensive strategy, so weigh it carefully. The following suggestions will maximize the benefits this option will offer you.

1. Have a concise presentation that you can adapt to varied conversations. Remember that you will be speaking to a large number of people in a short span of time, and make certain that your presentation is client-centered.
2. Keep a sign-up sheet handy, so that you can send a follow-up letter or make a follow-up phone call.
3. Have cards and brochures readily available, along with any other material that may help potential clients to understand what you do (articles you have published, etc.).
4. Use audiovisuals, such as posters or a short automatic slide presentation. Since you are unlikely to be able to spend much time with any one person, this is a good way of extending your contact.
5. Have your calendar ready so that you can make appointments for follow-up visits.
6. Follow up rapidly on those clients who express needs that your service can address.

Business Cards

Business cards are a good marketing investment. They are a convenient way of maintaining client awareness and maximizing invidual contacts. A client who has your business card is likely to pass it on to others who identify a need related to your services: "Oh, I met someone last week who works with those kinds of problems. Here's her card; maybe she can help you."

Remember that a business card must capture attention and describe what you do in a memorable way. Print style, phrasing, and logos should be carefully considered.

Brochures, Flyers, or Circulars

Brochures, flyers, and circulars provide more information than business cards do. They can increase client awareness and understanding and promote recognition of clients' needs. Moreover, they can be distributed in a variety of ways: as handouts, through the mail, or given to clients to pass on to others. Five guidelines should be kept in mind in the preparation of these materials.

1. Take a client-centered approach. Rather than focus solely on your services or skills, concentrate on clients' problems first, then discuss how your service will eliminate or modify these problems.
2. Include information about how to contact you.
3. Think about hiring an expert to help you with artwork and design.
4. Include information about your expertise.
5. Evaluate your return on this investment. How many clients do you get through this strategy? Is it worth the cost?

Mailings

Mailings increase market visibility and enhance client understanding, but they can be very expensive. Target your market carefully. Evaluate how much business the mailings generate, and base your subsequent use on this evaluation.

Advertising

Media advertising has several advantages: the ability to reach a wide audience, the opportunity to educate that audience, and the prestige that quality advertising can generate. The critical word is *quality*. As Cook (1980) notes,

> Good ads come through innovation and creativity spawned from deep commitment and total understanding of both product and market. Good advertising catches the spirit of the entrepreneur. It breaks new ground, seems fresh and different, provocative, and new. (p. 116)

The standards are high, and the strategy is expensive. To maximize your investment, consider hiring a professional to help you with your media advertising. Each of the media has its own advantages and disadvantages; a thoughtful comparison is essential.

1. Radio allows you to get close to your audience and explain your services. The potential audience is sizable, and you have a good chance of obtaining people's undivided attention if you reach them when they are alone.

2. Television has two advantages: a large audience and a multisensory impact, which captures audience attention. Effective use of TV, however, demands expertise and is costly.

3. Newspapers are perceived as a source of news; use of them lends credibility to your presentation. "Advertising in the newspaper is a powerful strategy that requires special skills. Expert marketing assistance can be very beneficial. (Levinson, 1984).

4. Journals have the advantage of greater reader involvement. This gives you the opportunity to educate and inform readers, because they are likely to "stay with you."

5. The Yellow Pages are used by prospects already interested in a service. Therefore, Yellow Pages advertising efforts should focus on how you are uniquely prepared to meet client's needs. The success of this strategy varies with the type of business, the likelihood that clients will recognize their needs, and the competition's name recognition factor. This strategy is best used in combination with others.

Advertising occasionally comes in the form of interviews by the local media. This free publicity has the added advantage of generating credibility. Stay alert to potential public relations opportunities of this sort.

Publications, Workshops, and Seminars

These methods can not only increase client awareness and understanding but also add to your credibility. Many nurse entrepreneurs have found them useful tools; however, several who have used these methods feel that they are not cost-effective, given that a considerable amount of time can be expended without attracting many clients. If marketing is your rationale for generating publications and presenting workshops and seminars, make certain that the increase in the number of clients justifies your choice.

We have reviewed the basic concepts that support a marketing process and discussed common promotional strategies. You must now integrate this information if you are to analyze your marketing needs correctly. Exercise 6.1 will help you to do this.

✓ Exercise 6.1 Market Information

Instructions. Complete this form for each of your client groups.

1. What is your client group?
2. What is your image with this Group? What is the source of this image? What do you plan to do to maintain or improve it?

Image	Cause	Strategy to Maintain or Improve

3. How would you describe your product? What are its unique features? How do clients perceive it?

4. What is the desired placement of your business in the market?

5. What is your pricing strategy? What will you charge for your service? Be explicit (cost per hour or unit of service).

How would you describe the competition? What is the unique factor that differentiates you from the competition?

6. What are your promotion strategies? Complete the following chart.

Promotion Strategies

Goal	Strategy	Cost per Month	Person Accountable

Once you obtain a clear picture of the market in in which you will operate, you are ready to develop a marketing plan.

THE MARKETING PLAN

Your marketing plan will include the following components (Kotler, 1986, p. 73):

- an executive summary,
- a table of contents,
- the current marketing situation,
- threats and opportunities,
- objectives and issues,
- marketing strategies,
- action programs,
- budgets, and
- controls.

Executive Summary

The executive summary briefly lists and describes the major goals and strategies covered in the marketing plan. It specifies the amount of sales targeted for the year and lists the percentage by which this amount is an increase over the previous year's sales. Moreover, it explains why you think it is possible to achieve this sales goal. It may, for example, be because of increased personnel or resources in your organization, or because of changes in the external environment, such as increased demand from customers or decreased competition from competitors.

The executive summary should also include a review of the finances necessary to achieve your objectives. The costs typically arise from advertising and sales promotion. They are frequently listed as percentages of projected sales; for example, the advertising budget may be $10,000 or 1 percent of the projected sales.

Table of Contents

As in any multiple-page document the table of contents tells the reader the location of specific parts of the plan.

Current Marketing Situation

The current marketing situation component provides information about the target market and how your company serves it. It covers four topics: market description, product review, competition, and distribution.

The market description section defines the target market, assesses its size, and describes its needs, and lists the circumstances that may have an impact on the target's purchasing behavior. If you are already making sales, the product review section describes the product/service you are selling, and lists the price and the gross margins. The competition section describes your competitor's strategies in regard to pricing, distribution, promotion, and quality; it also lists the market share of each competitor. The distribution section is important if you produce a product. It contains data on recent sales trends and developments in distribution.

Threats and Opportunities

The next component of the marketing plan is concerned with the threats and opportunities facing the product/service you sell. Day-to-day business activities often consume all of an entrepreneur's time. Understandably, you may tend to focus on present problems and concerns. Excessive focus on the present leads to tunnel vision, and the unfortunate result of such tunnel vision is that your future may be neglected, and you may either fail to take advantage of opportunities or neglect to defend yourself against threats.

The purpose of this component of the plan is to ensure that you build future considerations into your approach to business. Awareness of external events is the primary source of ideas about threats and opportunities. Among the events and conditions that may effect a nursing business are

- the nursing shortage;
- Federal interest in, legislation aimed at, and funds allocated for alleviating the shortage;
- the inability of nurse practitioners to obtain malpractice insurance;
- the increased acuity of hospitalized patients; and
- the rise of new classifications of health-care providers.

Depending on your perspective, any of these developments may represent a threat or an opportunity for your business. You must categorize and rank the effect an event will have on your business, then make plans to optimize the opportunity or neturalize the danger. If numerous threats and opportunities exist, it is essential that you determine what impact each of them will have on your business and how strong that impact will be.

Your plan must include strategies for eliminating those threats that are the most serious and the most likely to occur. Occurrences that have both a high probability and a high severity are the ones that necessitate a contingency plan. Your plan should also be able to assess opportunities for probability of success and attractiveness of the opportunity to the company. For opportunities that rank high in both regards, you should delineate how you intend to take advantage of the situation.

Objectives and Issues

In this component of the marketing plan, you establish objectives for the threats and opportunities you choose to address. The objectives you wish to achieve should be described in terms that are meaningful to the company—for example, the percentage increase in sales, the percentage increase in profit on sales, or the percentage increase in market share you wish to achieve. These objectives must then be evaluated. If, for instance, you wish to achieve a 50 percent pretax profit on sales but need 100 percent of the market to do that, you must consider certain issues. Two would be of particular importance. First, is it realistic to think that you can achieve 100 percent of the market share? Second, what other actions could you take to increase your pretax profit on sales by 50 percent without having to capture 100 percent of the market share? Could you drop products/services with a low profit margin and market lines with a high profit margin more heavily? Could you increase the prices on some lines? Could you decrease the expenses associated with producing your product/service?

Marketing Strategies

This component of the plan describes the methods by which you will attain the objectives you have established. There are three variables you can manipulate to accomplish your objectives: (1) target markets, (2) the marketing mix, and (3) the marketing budget.

Target Markets. Your strategies should be based on an understanding of which segments you can service best and how to appeal to these segments effectively. When more than one target market is involved, strategies must be specifically tailored to the special characteristics and needs of each of them.

Marketing Mix. The elements of the marketing mix include pricing, placement, and promotion of new or existing products/services. Each of these elements can be manipulated to achieve the balance that will lead to the fullest possible achievement of your objectives. As you manipulate these elements, consider and be able to explain how each of the strategies will be affected by the threats and opportunities you identified earlier in your marketing plan.

Budget. You should determine the amount of money to be spent on implementing market strategies by estimating the amount needed to achieve the best overall results for the company. Since money is a finite resource, you must balance the results you can achieve against the amount of money you are willing to spend to accomplish them.

Action Plan

The next component of the marketing plan, the action plan, explains how resources are allocated and provides a timetable for accomplishing the plan. It also states who will perform what activities, when, why, and how.

Budgets

The budget is organized so as to show how many new sales the marketing plan will generate and what profits, losses, or expenses are to be expected. The budget is the tool that regulates all decisions made in regard to the action plan.

Controls

The final component of the marketing plan has to do with the controls used to monitor progress. Usually, the controls are goals that are to be achieved within a specified period. Failure to achieve goals within the specified period necessitates the corrective action.

How complex your marketing plan should be depends on your particular business situation. If clients are knocking at the door and requesting your services before you even hang out a sign, or if referrals from previous clients are already generating a growing market, you may not need to develop a formal marketing plan. Most entrepreneurs, however, have to develop a plan that addresses marketing issues at some point in the life of their business. At times—for instance, when the market is highly competitive, when a product or service is untried, or when an entrepreneur has a neutral or negative public image—hiring a marketing specialist may be advisable. In many situations, however, entrepreneurs can use basic marketing skills, combined with creativity, to develop a winning market plan without any outside help. The information in this chapter can be used in a wide range of situations to analyze marketing problems, to develop marketing approaches for the early days, to prepare a basic marketing plan as your business status becomes more complex, or to use the services of an expert skillfully.

To get the most out of the following chapter, which deals with financing, you must have a solid working knowledge of the marketing process. Before proceeding to chapter 7, test your knowledge by completing the marketing section of the working copy business plan in appendix B. Even if you do not intend to use a formal business plan to obtain capital, a structured marketing process can help you to take advantage of any available opportunities for success.

7 FINANCING A BUSINESS

How much money is needed to start up a business varies tremendously, depending on the type of business. Considerable variation was noted among the nurses who responded to our survey, who did not make up a particularly large sample. In 50 responses to the question, "What were your original start-up costs?" the amounts needed for start-up ranged from less than $300 to $1.5 million. (see Table 7.1).

SOURCES OF START-UP FINANCING

Almost 60 percent of the nurse entrepreneurs who responded to the question started their businesses with $2,000 or less. The sources of money for the start-ups were personal funds, bank loans, and retainer fees. Forty-two of the nurses reported relying, at least to some extent, on their own funds. Thirteen took out bank loans, and two had retainers with clients.

Personal Funds

The most common source of start-up capital for any entrepreneur is personal funds, which includes salaries, savings, spouse's funds, and money

TABLE 7.1 Original Start-Up Costs for 50 Nurse Entrepreneurs

Start-Up Costs ($)	Nurses (N)
0–500	11
501–1,000	6
1,001–2,000	13
2,001–5,000	4
5,001–10,000	10
10,001–50,000	5
50,001–100,000	0
100,001–1,000,000	0
1,000,001–2,000,000	1

given to, loaned to, or invested in the business by family and friends. Investments may be one of two types: equity or debt. Someone who invests money in your business and becomes a part owner has an equity investment, which means that he or she is either a general partner, a limited partner, or a shareholder in your corporation. An investor who loans you money and expects to be paid back with interest has a debt investment.

The amount required for a start-up may be greater than the personal funds available to you. Before you look for additional financing, reexamine your assessment of needs and resources for the business. Look first at the financial section of your business plan. Is there anything that can be done to bring down the cost of producing your product/service? Is it possible to bring the breakeven point closer to the beginning of the business? Should you be renting equipment rather than buying it? Can you move up the date of the first expected sale?

Another likely area to investigate for additional resources is that of living expenses. Reevaluate your living expenses to determine if they can be decreased to make more cash available for the business. If after careful scrutiny, you still find that your requirements exceed your resources, the next logical step is to borrow money from a lending institution.

Borrowing Funds

The primary source of borrowed money is the bank. Although it is not always obvious, the money that you apply for from state and federal programs, loan companies, mortgage lenders, and small business investment companies ultimately comes from the bank.

Commercial banks supply over 65 percent of the capital requirements of small businesses (Silvester, 1984). There are numerous types of bank loans for which you can apply. Loans are typically described according to how long they are in effect. *Short-term* (or *operating*) loans usually extend for one year or less. These loans are a type of debt financing and are repaid in one lump payment. They are usually obtained for the purpose of financing inventory, accounts receivable, special purchases or promotions, and other items that require working capital during peak periods. If taking out a short-term loan is to work to your advantage, the loan should be paid back out of the returns earned on sales taking place within that peak period.

A *line of credit* is merely a particular form of short-term loan. It is a specified amount of money that you may use if the need arises. As a rule, it is established for a one-year period, after which time renegotiation may lead to renewal of the line. Credit lines may be either revolving or nonrevolving; the distinguishing feature of a revolving loan fund is that it increases as you need the money. Credit lines can often be obtained more quickly than a term loan. The interest rate fluctuates, but they may have a lower initial interest rate than a term loan, and they are available at most banks. Bank loans may be secured or unsecured; a secured loan is one that is backed by some asset to protect the lender against loss. The collateral used to secure a line of credit is your accounts receivable (the money owed to you by customers) and your inventory.

Intermediate-term loans are in effect for one to five years. These loans are used to purchase equipment or to provide working capital for a business that is growing rapidly.

Long-term loans extend for five years or more. These loans are often used to purchase or lease equipment; to buy real estate; to finance acquisitions, major plant expansions, or leveraged buyouts; or to supply working capital. Whether you should finance equipment with a long-term loan depends on how long the equipment is likely to last.

There are several simple steps you can take to improve your chances of getting a bank loan. First, since the bank is certain to want a copy of your business plan along with the loan application, anticipate this requirement and make sure that your business plan is up to date, clear, and concise.

Second, avoid the temptation to overstate your ability to repay loans or to exaggerate your profits, sales, or financial forecasts. If you are aware of problems in your business, be honest about them in talking to your banker. Trust is a vital element in this relationship: attempt at deception will hurt your chances more than would disclosing the element you sought to hide or disguise.

Third, when preparing for your appointment with the loan officer, think about your request from his or her perspective. Anticipate the loan officer's questions and concerns. Put together a comprehensive presentation detailing how much money is needed, how long it will be needed, how it will be spent, when it will be spent, and how the money will help your company be more profitable. Be able to specify how and when the money will be repaid, what the sources of repayment are, and what collateral you intend to use to secure the loan. In the course of your presentation, remember to ask the lender to give you a specific period of time within which you will know if your loan is granted or denied.

Since borrowing money takes time, you should start looking for money long before you actually need it. Your loan may be turned down in one institution, only to be granted in another, or it may be turned down by several. Remember that bankers frequently can offer good advice that you can use to make your loan application more acceptable or your request more appropriate. Always ask for their suggestions and recommendations. If your request is turned down, be sure you understand exactly why it was turned down and what you have to do to make the request acceptable.

You cannot know in advance exactly how a given bank will react to your request. Nurse entrepreneurs have had a wide range of experiences with banks, as the following remarks and anecdotes illustrate.

- "I had to submit eight proposals to get three accepted."
- "Be a man! It's a hell of a lot easier to get money."
- "I went to the first bank, met the VP in charge of loans, and first talked about my idea. Then I did a formal proposal and business plan, went to lunch with her, and refined the ideas. She investigated all sources of financing available to me and helped me through the application process. I found the bank very helpful."
- "It was very difficult; banks said I was high-risk." [The amount requested was $10,000.]
- "The original attempt at a line of credit wasn't successful: we were turned down by the bank. We succeeded with our second attempt."
- "We had no trouble getting a loan from the bank." [The amount requested was $20,000.]
- "The bank turned us down, but six months later we had a $50,000 line of credit."
- "We had an MBA develop a business plan. The banker was receptive, and we had good enough personal collateral." [The amount requested was $4,000.]
- "We had to use our incomes combined with our husbands' for that first loan." [The amount requested was between $1,000 and 2,000.]
- "My physician partner tried for a bank loan and was refused."
- "I applied for a business loan at no less than 12 banks and financial institutions. I had a very thorough and professionally prepared 17-page loan proposal, which I left at each place I applied, and I made appointments for follow-up to allow the bank officers adequate time for consideration and evaluation. When I retured to one bank, one older gentleman responsible for such decisions put his arm around my shoulders and told me, 'You would be better off asking for $10,000 to go to the Caribbean than to do this.'"

Banks are the main source of loans to entrepreneurs, and usually the first to be approached. They are not, however, the only source; alternative sources do exist.

Small Business Association

The Small Business Association has several financial assistance programs that may be of interest to the nurse entrepreneur. These programs provide funding that supports federally specified targets or objectives. (Since the guidelines change frequently, you should consult the SBA at about the time that you need to borrow money.) It is one of the stated goals of the SBA to assist entrepreneurs to start or expand their businesses, but this organization is often the entrepreneur's last resort for obtaining money. Typically, the SBA guarantees a loan with a commercial bank rather than makes a direct loan to your business. The loan guarantee is for 90 percent of the loan, up to $500,000. How much you are entitled to borrow is determined by how much business equity you have: three to five times your business equity is the amount the SBA will usually guarantee. The guaranteed loan protects the lender in the event that the entrepreneur defaults.

The first requirement for participating in the SBA program is that your loan request must have been rejected by private lenders. There are other requirements you must meet as well. Your company may not exceed the SBA standards for maximum size. (For service businesses, this is defined as annual sales not exceeding 2 to 8 million dollars; the precise limit is different for different types of service business.) Moreover, your company must be independently owned and operated, must comply with federal employment laws, must not dominate its field, and must not plan to use the money for speculation, lending, or investment or for the acquisition of real estate for sale or investment.

The process of applying for SBA assistance is complex and time consuming. You will need to have a business plan and a loan application. The SBA will scrutinize these and other documents carefully to determine if you are eligible for a loan guarantee. This process normally takes longer than the comparable processing in a bank would. If your banker is familiar with this application process, he or she can help you through the entire procedure.

Assistance in applying for SBA loans is also obtained through certain small business lending concerns that act like banks. The names and addresses of the organizations of this type in your area are available from the SBA, Financial Assistance Division, Office of Lender Relations, Non-Bank Lender Section, Washington, DC 20416.

Fewer than half of all SBA applications for a loan guarantee are approved (Fritz, 1987). Even if the SBA agrees to guarantee a loan for you, however, there are any number of reasons why lending institutions might be reluctant to loan you the money. If you are unable to get a loan guarantee, the SBA may offer to participate with the lender in providing the loan. Under this participation program, the lender must provide at least 25 percent of the loan, and the SBA provides the rest, up to $150,000. Your chances of getting money in this way are slim, since private lenders and the SBA rarely agree on the worthiness of any given application.

Yet another alternative is to apply for a direct loan from the SBA. If you are considering this approach, remember that there may be waiting lists for these direct loans, and loans of more than $150,000 are rarely given.

The Government Printing Office describes federal assistance programs in an annual publication called the *Catalog of Federal Domestic Assistance*. This publication is available from the Government Printing Office, Washington, DC.

State and Local Government Agencies

Most state and local governments are actively involved in enhancing the economic well-being of the areas under their jurisdiction. Consequently, most maintain programs that provide assistance of some type—financial, managerial, or other—to entrepreneurs. You can find out about programs of this type in your area by asking your banker, calling your local Chamber of Commerce, or calling your city or county administrator's office.

Foundations

You may be able to get a loan, a grant, or some other type of assistance from a foundation. Foundations give money to support projects that they deem worthy. They usually have a sphere of interest, such as health care–related projects, on which they focus. If the foundations in your area are not interested in the type of project you need funded, they should be able to suggest others that might be interested. Foundations usually do not limit their support to the geographic area in which they are located.

For information on foundations, your library should be your first resort. There are also additional sources of information about foundations that are open to the public without charge:

- The Foundation Center
888 Seventh Avenue
New York, NY 10019
- The Foundation Center
10001 Connecticut Avenue NW
Washington, DC 20036
- Donors' Forum
208 LaSalle Street
Chicago, IL 60654

Venture Capital

Venture capital firms are backed by the combined resources of many wealthy investors who wish to invest in small business. Money obtained from venture capital firms usually takes the form of an equity investment; that is, the venture capitalist becomes part owner of your company.

Venture capitalists are attracted by the prospect of fast growth: they expect their original investment to grow 500 percent within three years or 1,000 percent within five years (Silvester, 1987). Other features that are likely to attract the interest of venture capitalists are:

- a management team with an impressive track record of success,
- the intention to expand the business to a substantial size,
- a well-thought-out business plan with five-year financial projections, and
- willingness to permit investors to get out with their gains in five to eight years, whether by going public, by selling out later, or by sharing ownership.

Some venture capital funds focus on investments in specific sectors. The minimum and maximum amounts of money available for investment in a given project are often predetermined as well. Thus, you need information about specific venture capital funds before you can determine which ones are appropriate for your purposes. The National Venture Capital Association, 1655 North Fort Myer Drive, Suite 700, Arlington, VA, 22209, can supply you with a list of venture capitalists that specifies the information you most need to know about a given fund.

SBICs and MESBICs

The Small Business Association is also involved with venture capital. Specifically, it licenses small business investment corporations (SBICs) and minority enterprise small business investment corporations (MESBICs). An SBIC can borrow up to four times the amount of capital it has invested from the US Treasury. It then lends out these funds and attempts to make a profit on each loan transaction. As a rule, SBIC loans are given to provide equity capital, long-term loans, and management assistance to small businesses. Businesses that are at least one year old are more attractive to SBICs than newer businesses. The minimum investment is about $100,000; the maximum is $2 to $3 million in long-term financing. There are about 400 SBICs across the country. You may obtain a listing from the National Association of Small Business Investment Companies, 618 Washington Building, Washington, DC 20005.

The MESBICs deal strictly with minority-owned businesses. They offer different financing options and operate under different constraints than the SBICs do.

National Center for Nursing Research—Public Health Service

The National Center for Nursing Research (NCNR) is another source of funds that nurses should investigate. There are specific guidelines for funding areas, and there is an increasing interest in innovative practice options. The Public Health Service also has a Small Business Innovation Research (SBIR) program. Since the NCNR is part of the PHS, contacting the NCNR first is likely to provide you with additional information.

Write to the National Center for Nursing Research, National Institute of Health, Building 38A, Room B2E17, Bethesda, MD 20894, (301) 496-0526.

Any source you approach in your search for business money is interested primarily in how good a financial risk you are, though of course the source will also have to analyze your business plan carefully and evaluate your business acumen. Exercise 7.1 contains a checklist that will help you to anticipate how a lender will assess this aspect of your personal history.

✓ Exercise 7.1 Financial Risk Checklist: Are You a Good Financial Risk?

Instructions. Place a check on the line next to the correct answer to each question.

1. Why do you need the money?
   - To expand the business _____ 10 points
   - To operate the business _____ 5 points
   - To start a business _____ 0 points

2. How long have you been in business?
   - Three years or more _____ 10 points
   - One to three years _____ 5 points
   - Just beginning _____ 0 points

3. Does the business have a good financial history and good prospects for continued profitability?
   - Strong history/outlook _____ 10 points
   - Steady history/outlook _____ 5 points
   - Inconsistent history, no history, history of losses, or poor history _____ 0 points

4. What is the business's profitability and return on investment compared to the industry average?
   - Above average ______ 10 points
   - Average ______ 5 points
   - Below average ______ 0 points

5. Divide the business's current assets by its liabilities. How does this ratio compare to the industry average?
   - Above average ______ 10 points
   - Average ______ 5 points
   - Below average ______ 0 points

6. Do you have established banking/funding sources?
   - Several ______ 10 points
   - My local bank ______ 5 points
   - No ______ 0 points

7. Are you well known in the community?
   - Widely known ______ 10 points
   - Somewhat known ______ 5 points
   - No ______ 0 points

8. How are your personal and business credit ratings?
   - Good to excellent ______ 10 points
   - Fair ______ 5 points
   - Poor or unrated ______ 0 points

9. Do you have a business plan?
   - Formally prepared and documented ______ 10 points
   - Informally prepared or documented ______ 5 points
   - No ______ 0 points

10. How are your controls over finances and internal accounting?
    - Good to excellent ______ 10 points
    - Weak in some areas ______ 5 points
    - Poor or nonexistent ______ 0 points

11. Do you have sufficient business insurance?
    - Yes, including key man insurance ______ 10 points
    - Generally good ______ 5 points
    - No ______ 0 points

12. Of the key functions in your business—here considered to be administration, policy, marketing, finance, personnel, and production—how many do you handle yourself?
    Two ______ 10 points
    Three or four ______ 5 points
    Five or all ______ 0 points

13. How would someone evaluate your employees' competence, experience, and loyalty?
    Above average ______ 10 points
    Average ______ 5 points
    Below average ______ 0 points

Scoring. If you score 100 or more points on this analysis, you should be able to get the funds that you need at a reasonable cost. If you score 50 to 99 points, it will help to have good connections with the lender. Can you improve in any of the areas on which you scored poorly? If you scored fewer than 50 points, you will definitely find it difficult to locate funds.

Adapted from Fritz, 1987. Used with permission

If your financial risk score is low, work on your problem areas before you meet with a potential lender. You may have to improve your presentation of the success potential of your business idea, find more collateral for a loan, or obtain your first contract before any money is forthcoming. Remember to check out the variety of avenues open to you. Tables 7.2 and 7.3 list a number of sources of asset and debt funding that you should consider.

So far, we have discussed finances in terms of the money you need to start your business. Eventually, however, you will have to familiarize yourself with other aspects of the topic. If you are to be a successful entrepreneur, you will need to know how to manage and keep track of the money you obtain.

MANAGING BUSINESS FINANCES

Some new entrepreneurs shudder at the thought of the financial maze that awaits them and are tempted to turn the management of their business finances over to an accountant. There are three important reasons why you should not do this, even if you have an accountant available.

TABLE 7.2 Requirements for Asset-Based Lending

Variables	Receivables	Inventory	Machine and Equipment (M&E)	Real Estate
Amount as % of qualifying collateral	80–90%	15–75%	50–100%	50–70%
Qualifying collateral	Current receivables (customary dated terms considered current) less than 60 or 90 days old; reduced by estimated returns, allowances, or other setoffs; reduced by large, concentrated accounts (evaluated separately); reduced by historical bad debts experience; excludes most related party and foreign accounts (evaluated separately)	Variables by specialty vs commodity nature; higher %s are for commodity-type items; work in process is generally excluded; highest % for finished goods; lending base is set at a quick liquidation value; as is, lending percentage generally averages 40–60% of cost.	Lower %s for used or specialty M&E; higher %s for newer or commodity-type M&E values are quick liquidation realizable values which may be 50% or less of an in-place, in-use appraisal	Lower %s for special purpose facilities; may be based on quick liquidation appraisal

continued

TABLE 7.2 (cont.)

Variables	Receivables	Inventory	Machine and Equipment (M&E)	Real Estate
Loan structure	Revolving credit (1–3 years)	Revolving credit or term line (1–3 years)	Term loans: 3–5 years; longer in certain cases	Term varies; rarely beyond 10–15 years.
Other provisions	Approval of new accounts; cash collections are deposited to an account controlled by lender; deposits credited against loan within an agreed-upon processing period (delays are a hidden loan cost); loan advances made on request up to available collateral; both the lender and borrower maintain receivable records that must be periodically reconciled; verification of shipments and orders	Security and insurance provisions; adequate inventory accounting systems required (perpetural inventories); verification of orders, receipts, and usage (withdrawal); periodic reconciliation with lender usually done in conjunction with receivable line and related customer cash-processing procedures	Security, maintenance, and insurance provisions; adequate inventory type records and identification systems; possible restrictions on leasing to others; amortizing by periodic payments	Standard mortgage provisions; may be fully amortizing or with balloon payment at end; will consider construction loans

TABLE 7.2 (cont.)

Variables	Receivables	Inventory	Machine and Equipment (M&E)	Real Estate
Approval and monitoring process	Approval requires a lender's audit of account balances, shipping and processing procedures, confirmation; operational-type audits of several management information system areas; monitoring requires periodic surprise lender's audits, continuous document verification, and periodic confirmation	Approval requires a lender's audit of inventories, receiving and production records, operational-type audits of management information systems, inventory security, etc.; appraisals possible; monitoring requires periodic surprise lender's audits, and continuous document verification	Approval requires a lender's appraisal; monitoring requires periodic surprise lender's audit and possible confirmation of insurance and maintenance agreements	Approval requires appraisals and general credit approval; monitoring is by periodic credit reviews and inspection audits
Costs	Floating prime + 2–6 points, audit fees, usage and nonusage line fees of 1–2 points	Floating prime + 2–6 points; audit and commitment fees	Floating prime + 2–6 points; audit and commitment fees	Floating prime + 2–6 points; audit and commitment fees

Adapted from Fritz, 1984, pp. 80–81. Used with permission.

TABLE 7.3 Sources of Debt Funding

Variables	Commercial Banks	Savings & Loan Associations	Commercial Finance Companies (Asset-Based Lenders)	Leasing Companies	Government-Assisted Sources	Industrial Revenue Bonds
Loan Types						
Demand	Frequent	Occasional	Rare		Rare	
Short term (5 years or less)	Frequent	Occasional	Occasional	Operating and financing leases	Frequent	
Intermediate (5–15 years)	Occasionally up to 10 years	Occasional	Occasional	Operating and financing leases	Frequent	Frequent (sale-lease backs)
Long-term (over 15 years)	Rare	Frequent	Occasional	Operating and financing leases	Occasional	Frequent (sale-lease backs)
Uses						
Revolving credit	Occasional	Rare	Frequent		Occasional	
Working Capital	Frequent	Occasional	Frequent		Frequent	
Growth capital: Machinery and equipment	Frequent	Occasional	Frequent	Frequent	Frequent	Frequent
Real estate	Occasional	Frequent	Occasional	Frequent	Occasional	Frequent

Acquisitions or general expansion	Occasional	Rare	Frequent	Occasional	Occasional	Occasional (expansion not acquisition)
Risk capital	Rare	Rare	Rare		Occasional to frequent (varies by provider)	
Amounts available	Varies by institution	Varies by institution	Varies by collateral provided	Varies by asset leased	Varies by provider (usually less than $1,000,000)	Varies by issuer and user
Interest rate base	Prime rate plus 1.4 points	Long-term AAA or government bonds indices plus risk premiums (varying according to circumstances)	Prime plus 2 to 6 points	Prime plus 2 to 6 points	Varies by provider. SBA debentures or other government securities	Tax-free government bonds yields of issuer
Other terms						
Covenants						
Affirmative	Occasional	Frequent	Frequent	Only as to leased asset	Always	Always
Negative	Occasional	Frequent	Frequent	Only as to leased asset	Always	Always
Guarantees	Frequent	Frequent	Frequent	Occasional	Frequent	Generally
Security	Frequent	Frequent	Always	Title retained	Frequent	Always

continued

TABLE 7.3 (cont.)

Other	Varies by loan type	Fees and other costs; extensive default provisions	Fees and other costs	Provisions on taxes, insurance, and maintenance	Can have extensive public policy requirements	Very extensive tax and regulatory compliance provisions
Financial statements	Audited preferred	Audited preferred	Audited preferred	Audited preferred	Audited preferred	Audited preferred
Request documents	Generally not complex; more detail required for longer terms; varies at times by security	Generally not complex, but requires extensive appraisals of securing assets	Generally not complex, but requires extensive supporting documents and appraisals of some securing assets: significant preparation aid furnished	Generally not complex; varies in circum-stances	Complex and extensive, significant preparation aid may be provided	Complex and extensive, significant legal and tax compliance documentation
Borrower stage of development:						
Start-up	Occasionally with guarantees	Infrequent	Infrequent	Frequent	Frequent	Occasional

Adapted from Fritz, 1984, pp. 87–89. Used with permission.

1. An understanding of the financial risks of doing business is a critical element of many start-up decisions. An entrepreneur who lacks this understanding is likely to make choices that jeopardize his or her chances of success.

2. Any entrepreneur who needs to obtain money for a business venture must be able to demonstrate to potential lenders that he or she has an in-depth awareness of the financial implications of all business activity.

3. Financial performance is intrinsically related to growth and survival. An entrepreneur who does not have a firm grasp of financial performance measures cannot plan strategically or evaluate progress effectively.

The key tools for understanding, planning, and monitoring financial activity are seven essential documents that supply information about your personal and business financial status: (1) the personal financial statement, (2) the budget, (3) the budget deviation analysis, (4) the balance sheet, (5) the income statement, (6) the cash flow schedule, and (7) the break-even analysis. These documents are an important part of the initial business plan and act as an ongoing financial monitoring system. They exist in a variety of formats. This section contains a sample of each document and gives examples of how to use them. You need not adhere strictly to these samples, however; you may choose to alter them to suit your special needs, to develop your own variants, or to obtain other forms from your accountant or financial advisor.

The forms you select should provide information that you can understand and use. If you are working with an accountant, ask for an explanation of the information and an analysis of how it affects your business decisions. Each document, except for the personal financial statement, depicts a specific part of the financial activity of your business; they should all be reviewed together at frequent intervals. The personal financial statement is prepared at start-up and whenever significant business changes necessitate reevaluation of your personal financial status.

Personal Financial Statement

The personal financial statement must be completed for each owner, partner, and stockholder owning 20 percent or more of the business. The form reproduced in Exercise 7.2 is similar to the forms most banks will ask you to complete when you apply for a business loan. Besides helping the bank assess your potential risk, completing this form enables you to answer the following questions.

1. Equity: How much money will you invest in the business start-up personally, and what is the source of these funds (self, family, friends)?
2. Collateral: What are you willing to lose to the lender if your business fails (house, property, etc.)?
3. Living expenses: What are your monthly living expenses? How will you survive until your business profits provide an adequate personal income? Most entrepreneurs estimate that you need at least one to two years of living expenses on hand if you intend to devote yourself full-time to the business.

✔ Exercise 7.2 Personal Financial Statement

Instructions. Complete the sample personal financial statement on pages 191–193 and answer the following questions.

1. What will you invest in the business?

Amount of Money	Source

2. What collateral will you provide?

Item	Appraised Value

3. What are your personal monthly expenses and how will you meet these costs?

Expenses	Strategy for Meeting Costs

Sample Personal Financial Statement

Personal

Name ______________________________

Address ______________________________

Assets	Indiv.	Joint	If joint w/ whom	Liabilities	Indiv.	Joint	If joint w/ whom
Cash on hand and in banks				Notes payable to banks—secured			
				—unsecured			
U.S. Government securities				Notes payable to relatives			
Listed securities							
Unlisted securities				Notes payable to others			
Mortgages owned							
Accounts and notes receivable due from relatives and friends				Accounts and bills due			
				Accrued interest, etc.			
Accounts and notes receivable due from others—good				Taxes unpaid or accrued			
—doubtful				Mortgages payable on real estate			
Real estate owned				Chattel mortgages and other liens payable			
Cash value life insurance				Other debts—itemize			
Automobiles							
Personal property							
Other assets—itemize							
				TOTAL LIABILITIES			
				Net Worth			
TOTAL ASSETS				TOTAL LIABILITIES AND NET WORTH			

Source of Income

Alimony, child support or maintenance income need not be revealed if you do not wish it to be considered as a basis for repaying this obligation.

	Indiv.	Joint	If joint w/ whom
Salary			
Bonds and commissions			
Dividends and bond interest			
Real estate income			
Other income—itemize			
TOTAL			

Personal Information

If you are applying for individual credit, information about your spouse or ex-spouse need not be revealed unless you are relying on income from alimony, child support or maintenance or on the income or assets of another person as a basis for repaying this obligation:

____

Business or occupation:

Partner or officer in other venture:

MARITAL STATUS (Do not complete if this is submitted for individual unsecured credit.)	No. of Dependents
☐ Married ☐ Separated ☐ Unmarried (including single, divorced or widowed)	

Contingent Liabilities

	Indiv.	Joint	If joint w/ whom
As endorser or co-maker.			
On leases or contracts			
Legal claims.			
Taxes not shown above: Income taxes			
Delinquent or contested taxes. . . .			
OTHER SPECIAL DEBTS.			

General Information

Are any assets pledged? ____________

Are you defendant in any suit or legal action?

____

Personal bank accounts carried at:

Individual: ____________

Joint: ____________

If joint, with whom: ____________

Have you ever taken bankruptcy? If yes, explain: ____________

____

List of Banks and Finance Companies Where Credit Has Been Obtained

Name(s) in Which Obtained	Name of Bank or Company	High Credit	Present Balance	Type of Loan

Remarks ______________________________

____

____

____

US Government and Listed Stocks and Bonds

Held in Name(s) of	Description	Cost	Market Value

Mortgages, Unlisted Securities and Other Investments

Held in Name(s) of	Description, Including Maturities	Cost	Market Value

Real Estate Owned

Description and Location	Title in Name(s) of	Market Value	Mortgages	Taxes Paid to

Life Insurance

Owner	Name of Company	Beneficiary	Amount	Cash Value	Loans

Accounts and Notes Receivables

Owner(s)	Debtor and Address	Present Balance Due

Personal Property and Vehicles

Description and Location	Owner(s)		Mortgages

The forgoing financial statement and explanations have been fairly and correctly presented according to the best of my knowledge and belief.

Date signed:__________________, 19____ Signature:________________________

Date signed:__________________, 19____ Signature:________________________

Reviewing your personal financial status is the first step in evaluating the overall financial implications of a business venture. The next six documents are concerned with your business rather than your personal finances. They portray the projected and actual flow of cash and other assets in the business.

Budget

Like the other documents considered in this section, the budget is both a planning tool and a control mechanism for the company's financial performance. As a planning tool, it requires you to make projections about the amount of income you will generate and the expenses you will incur. As a control device, the budget allows you to measure your actual financial performance against your projections through the use of a budget deviation report. A budget deviation report, reviewed monthly, helps you to eliminate costs that are out of line or alter your marketing strategies if sales fall below projected levels. The sample budget outlined in Exercise 7.3 includes items that constitute usual business expenses. You may want to add or delete certain items, depending on the specific needs of your business. To complete this exercise, you will need to review your answers to Exercises 5.1 and 5.2.

✔ Exercise 7.3 Company Budget

Instructions. On the chart that follows, project your monthly sales by estimating the units of service or products you plan to provide to clients each month. Next, if you are selling a product, list the cost of goods sold, which is the amount you paid for your inventory in order to have something to sell, directly under projected sales. Finally, project monthly expenses by dividing fixed costs (like rent) by 12 months, by placing costs in the month in which they occur (for instance, license renewal fees that are due each September would be placed under that month), or by estimating varying costs that vary by determining when they are most likely to occur (for instance, if you plan to attend your specialty convention, in what month is it usually held?).

	Start-Up	Month 1	2	3	4	5	6	7	8	9	10	11	12	Annual
Projected sales														
Cost of sales (minus)														
GROSS PROFIT														
Project costs														
Advertising														
Audiovisual														
Automobile														
Books														
Continuing education														
Depreciation														
Donations														
Dues/subscriptions														
Educational supplies														
Equipment														
Furniture														
Insurance—malpractice														
Insurance—life														
Insurance—health														
Insurance—disability														
Insurance—key person														
Interest														
Legal and accounting														
Office supplies														
Purchased services														

Exercise 7.3 (cont.)

		Month												
	Start-Up	1	2	3	4	5	6	7	8	9	10	11	12	Annual
Rent														
Repairs														
Salaries														
Taxes and license														
Taxes—payroll														
Telephone														
Travel														
TOTAL														
PROFIT (subtract total expenses from gross profit)														

This budget is your financial plan for the start-up period and the first year of operation. Using this information, you should be able to answer the following three questions and estimate the amount of capital necessary for your start-up.

1. How much money do you need to start your business and stay in operation before you begin to make a profit?
2. How much money will you invest? Subtract your answer to question 1 from your answer to question 2.
3. How much money do you need to borrow.

Budget Deviation Analysis

The budget is developed annually and is a statement of the financial goals for your company. To evaluate your actual financial performance, you must formulate a budget deviation statement and review it on a monthly basis. You can develop your own form, use an existing one, or obtain a computer printout if you have a computer. Your secretary can also prepare the form for your monthly review. Figure 7.1 is an example of a budget deviation statement form.

To utilize a budget variance analysis effectively, determine what percentage of variance suggests unacceptable performance. Then analyze any deviations monthly to identify causes of the variance and select remedies.

When you have prepared the budget, you have set in motion a basic financial review process. The last four of the seven essential documents represent distinct aspects of that process.

Balance Sheet and Income Statement

The balance sheet gives you a picture of how your business is doing at a specific point in time. Figures 7.2, 7.3, and 7.4 are provided to help you complete a balance sheet, illustrate the proper use of balance sheets and income statements. They reflect the first six months of a fictitious nurse-run company, Critical Care Educational Enterprises, whose equally fictitious proprietor is Jane Smith, RN.

Jane Smith has decided to start a business providing continuing education for critical care nurses. Fortunately, she just inherited $35,000 from an uncle, which she will invest as capital in the business. Since as a teacher she has a special interest in the utilization of high-tech equipment and monitoring devices and in the interpretation of and nursing responses to

Budget Deviation Analysis

Company name: ____________________ Month_______________ 19 ___

P = project amount; **A** = actual amount; **V** = variance amount

	Monthly Analysis			Year-to-Date Analysis		
Item	P	A	V	P	A	V
Projected sales						
Cost of sales						
GROSS PROFIT						
Projected costs						
Advertising						
Audiovisual						
Automobile						
Books						
Continuing education						
Depreciation						
Donations						
Dues/subscriptions						
Equipment						
Furniture						
Insurance—malpractice						
Insurance—life						
Insurance—health disability key person						
Interest						
Legal and accounting						
Office supplies						
Purchased services						
Rent						
Repairs						
Salaries						
Taxes and license						
Taxes—payroll						
Telephone						
Travel						
TOTAL						
PROFIT						

Figure 7.1 A sample budget deviation analysis form.

Figure 7.1 (cont.)

Comments (explain any variance of more than ____%):

Item#	Explanation of Variance

data derived from such equipment, she purchased simulators to use as learning aids. She also bought a home computer for the business. The total cost of this equipment was $15,000. She did not want to use her cash until she began to make a profit, so she used a $10,000 bank loan and $5,000 credit from her suppliers to pay for the equipment. Since she is selling a service rather than a product, she did not have to purchase an inventory. Her start-up balance sheet is shown in Figure 7.2.

During the first six months, Jane was very successful. She contracted for $35,000 worth of business and collected all but $5,000 of that amount. Her

Balance Sheet for Critical Care Educational Enterprises: Start-Up Period

1. **Assets** (what Jane has)	
Cash	$35,000
Accounts receivable	0
Equipment/buildings	15,000
TOTAL ASSETS	$50,000
2. **Liabilities** (what Jane owes)	
Accounts payable	$5,000
Bank loan	10,000
TOTAL LIABILITIES	$15,000
3. **Equity** (What is left that belongs to Jane)	
Capital	$35,000
Retained earnings*	0
TOTAL EQUITY	$35,000
TOTAL EQUITY AND LIABILITIES	$50,000

*This figure would be obtained from the income statement if Jane was already doing business.

Figure 7.2 An example of a balance sheet for a business in its start-up period.

income statement for this period (see Figure 7.3) reflects her business costs and her net profit. In the six-month balance sheet in Figure 7.4, the $30,000 in collected payments was used to pay the suppliers $2,000 and reduce the bank loan by $2,000. Jane also paid the $8,000 in operating costs reflected in the income statement, leaving $18,000 that was added to the cash assets. Her business equity reflects her original $35,000 investment and her net profit from the six-month period.

As Jane's company expands, other assets besides inventory, furniture, and equipment—such as: automobiles, investments, deposits, real estate, or land—maybe added to the list. Depreciation of equipment and other assets will also affect total assets. If Jane had sold shares in her business, the balance sheet would show stockholder's equity. Remember that the balance sheet portrays the company's worth at a single point in time; an income statement is necessary to explain changes in the company's assets from one period to another.

Now that you have studied the use of balance sheets and an income statement in a fictitious business, apply your knowledge to your own business by completing Exercises 7.4 and 7.5.

✔ Exercise 7.4 Start-up Balance Sheet

Instructions. Complete the form below using your start-up projections.

1. **Assets**

   Cash
   Accounts Receivable
   Equipment/Buildings
   TOTAL ASSETS

2. **Liabilities**

   Accounts payable
   Bank loan
   TOTAL LIABILITIES

3. **Equity**

   Capital
   Retained earnings
   TOTAL EQUITY
   TOTAL EQUITY AND LIABILITIES

Income Statement for Critical Care Educational Enterprises: First 6 Months

Sales	$35,000
(minus costs of goods sold*)	(0)
Gross profit	35,000
(minus expenses)	(8,000)
NET PROFIT (to retained earnings)	$27,000

*If Jane were selling a product, she would have had to purchase inventory in order to have something to sell. The cost of that inventory would have been reflected in the costs of goods sold.

Figure 7.3 An example of an income statement for a business in its first 6 months of operation.

Balance Sheet for Critical Care Educational Enterprises: First 6 Months

1. Assets	
Cash	$53,000
Accounts receivable	5,000
Inventory	0
Equipment and buildings	$15,000
TOTAL ASSETS	$73,000
2. Liabilities	
Accounts payable	$3,000
Bank loan	8,000
Other debts	0
TOTAL LIABILITIES	$11,000
3. Equity	
Capital	$35,000
Retained earnings	27,000
TOTAL EQUITY	$62,000
TOTAL EQUITY AND LIABILITIES	$73,000

Figure 7.4 An example of a balance sheet for a business after its first 6 months of operation.

✓ Exercise 7.5 Income Statement (Projection)

Instructions. Prepare an income projection for the first six months on the form below.

Sales	
(minus costs of goods sold)	( )
Gross profit	
(minus expenses)	( )
NET PROFIT	

The balance sheet and income statement alone do not provide a comprehensive view of how the business finances are being managed: they must be augmented by a cash flow schedule.

Cash Flow Schedule

This schedule traces "the impact of operations, as shown in the income statement, upon the cash account in order to try to maintain an adequate cash balance for payment of bills at all times" (Edmunds, 1982, p. 28). To make sound financial decisions and remain solvent, you must be able to project cash receipts and cash expenses on a month-to-month basis and evaluate your actual cash flow performance monthly. The cash flow schedule is a necessary tool for such projection and evaluation. Exercise 7.6 gives you the opportunity to develop a cash flow projection for your business.

✓ Exercise 7.6 Developing a Cash Flow Schedule

Instructions. On the form below, provide cash flow and cash expense estimates for your start-up date and for the first three months of operations. If your business is currently in operation, complete the schedule for the next three months. Add other items to the list as necessary.

The cash flow schedule is a control system that ensures that financial outcomes meet expected financial performance criteria. The information you receive from this form will tell you if there is enough cash to cover expenses, if you are meeting your financial goals, and if your break-even analysis was accurate.

Item	Start-Up		Month					
			1		2		3	
	Estimate	Actual	Estimate	Actual	Estimate	Actual	Estimate	Actual
Cash on hand, first of month or start-up								
Cash receipts								
Cash sales								
Accounts receivable								
Sales of assets								
Loans								
TOTAL								
Cash expenses								
Merchandise								
Equipment								
Payroll								
Operating expenses								
Purchasing of assets								
TOTAL								
Cash, end of month								

Break-Even Analysis

The break-even analysis is an estimate of the point at which a business becomes profitable—that is, the point at which the money received from the sale of the product or provision of a service exceeds the fixed and variable expenses of doing business. A break-even analysis is a necessary part of the business plan, but it can also help you with decisions related to expansion of business volume or addition of new product lines.

To formulate a break-even analysis, first list your fixed and variable expense projections and identify your cash revenue from each client sale, then determine how many sales are necessary before your income surpasses your fixed and variable expenses.

Examination of how a break-even analysis might be determined for the fictitious business described earlier should illustrate the value of this process. Jane Smith considers her unit of service to be a workshop hour, for which she charges $50. How many workshop hours will she need to provide in order to reach the break-even point? In order to answer that question, she first lists her fixed and variable expenses (see Figure 7.5). Fixed expenses are those that remain the same over time, regardless of the volume of sales; variable expenses are those that change in proportion to the sales volume. Her fixed expenses include rent, utilities, depreciation of equipment, and interest on loans and taxes, and her variable expenses for each eight-hour program include marketing, supplies, typing and copying of program materials (a purchased service), and travel.

The information in Figure 7.5 is plotted then on a break-even chart, as is shown in Figure 7.6, to provide a graphic display of Jane's break-even point. Expenses are indicated on the vertical scale and workshop contact hours

Annual Fixed Expenses		Variable Expenses per 8-Hour Program	
Rent	$ 3,600	Marketing	$30
Utilities	1,200	Supplies	12
Depreciation	1,500	Typing/ copying	35
Interest	1,700	Travel	22
Taxes	2,000		
TOTAL	$10,000	TOTAL	$99
		TOTAL PER 1 HOUR = $12.35	

Figure 7.5 Examples of fixed and variable expenses for a nurse-run business.

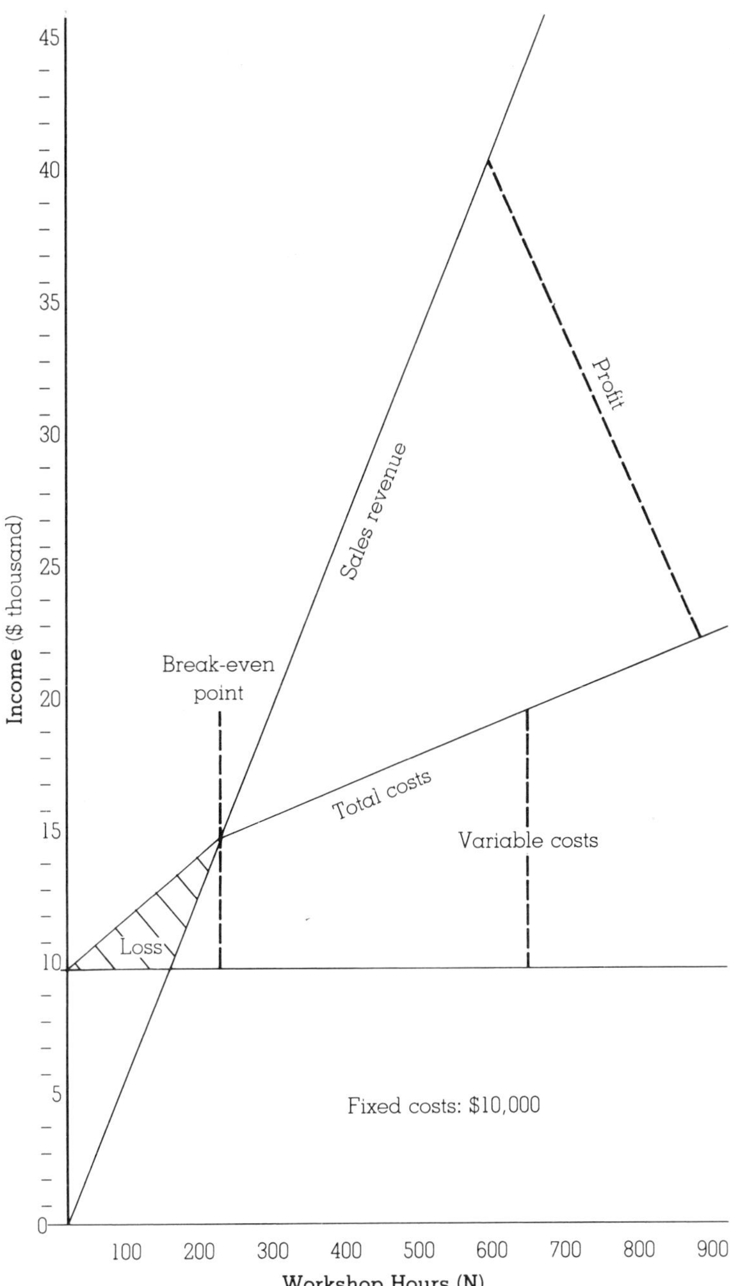

Figure 7.6 Example of a break-even chart on which the results of a break-even analysis are plotted.

on the horizontal scale. The $10,000 fixed cost is plotted as a horizontal line at the base of the chart, since it does not vary with the volume of activity. The variable cost is added to the fixed cost at the rate of approximately $12.35 per hour, which yields the ascending total costs per unit line. The sales revenue line is plotted diagonally from the lower left corner to the upper right corner. The break-even point is the point at which the revenue and total cost lines intersect. Jane's break-even point is about 230 hours. Beyond this point, all earnings represent profits unless the fixed or variable expenses change.

As Jane reviews this chart, she discovers that her profit after 900 workshop hours is about $25,000. Considering the amount of time she spends preparing for these classes, she has to ask herself, "Am I making a reasonable profit?" It is clear that Jane should think about options for lowering her break-even point and increasing her profits, such as reducing her costs and raising her prices. Like Jane, you can use this information in several ways: to determine if losses are likely to occur because of an increase in fixed costs and thus in the break even point; to decide whether the profit spread can be improved by raising prices or cutting costs; or to analyze how expansion will change fixed costs, increase variable costs, and alter the break-even analysis. Exercise 7.7 will help you establish a break-even point for your new business.

✔ Exercise 7.7 Break-Even Analysis

Instructions. Answer the following questions using information you have obtained about your business.

1. What is your unit of activity?

2. What is your price for each unit of activity?

3. What are your fixed and variable costs?

Fixed Costs	Variable Costs
TOTAL FIXED COSTS	TOTAL VARIABLE COSTS PER UNIT OF ACTIVITY

4. Plot your analysis on a graph below.

5. What is your break-even point? What changes could you make to create a more favorable break-even point?

The financial exercises in this chapter have two purposes. First, they are designed to prepare you to develop the necessary financial doucmentation for a business plan. Second, they are presented as planning tools that you need if you are to avoid the financial mistakes entrepreneurs frequently make.

COMMON FINANCIAL MISTAKES

Small businesses fail or get into financial trouble for a number of reasons. The following are the most common ones.

Running Out of Cash

Running out of cash is the most frequent cause of failure. It usually happens when the entrepreneur tries to expand too rapidly without regard to the amount of cash on hand to cover liabilities. Careful monitoring of current and projected cash flow relative to liabilities is essential. Remember, "cash and receivables should at least equal current liabilities, and current assets should at least be double current debts" (Edmunds, 1982, p. 43).

Failure to Use Profits

Letting profits gather dust is another pitfall to avoid. Profits above the needs of the business should be used for expansion or invested to create further assets. Knowing where your money is and how it can best be used is a prerequisite for financial growth. A financial advisor is a genuine asset when profits exceed necessary business expenses and liabilities.

Allowing Buildup of Accounts Receivable

Delinquent accounts mean that you are sharing your potential profits with your client. To return those profits to where they belong—in your business—pay attention to the collection process. Mail out statements promptly, and send reminders when payments are overdue. Some entrepreneurs have found it helpful to include payment specifics and describe delinquent payment policy in the contract.

Underpricing Product/Service

Nursers frequently underestimate the worth of their services, perhaps because of their professional socialization. Review your break-even point to determine whether your pricing structure is suitable. Remember that too low a price encourages potential clients to undervalue the quality of your service. Evaluate the market, and reassess your price structure frequently.

Forgettting to Pay Yourself

Unbelievable as it sounds, some entrepreneurs forget to establish and pay themselves a salary out of their business profits. Since the amount of the salary you pay yourself can affect your taxes, you should consult your accountant before making this decision.

The best strategy for avoiding the financial traps that exist is a simple one: develop the essential financial systems and forms, and evaluate your financial picture on a monthly basis. Goldstein (1985) estimates that "it will take 122 minutes of your time each month to monitor the results of your company's activity and give you a better understanding of your successes and/or failures. You will build a better business and make more money (p. 136). Your working knowledge of the finances of your business ensures that you are in control of its survival, improves your ability to use the expertise of your financial advisor wisely, and enables you to develop a business plan that is likely to interest potential sources of capital. One use for the information acquired in this is to help you write a business plan. Accordingly, turn to the working copy of the business plan in appendix B and complete the "selected financial information" section. Then proceed to chapter 8, where we consider the challenge that follows the start-up period: *survival.*

8 SURVIVAL AND GROWTH

When you are engrossed in your start-up activities, you are likely to put thoughts of survival and growth on the back burner, at least for the moment. This is a normal response and a harmless one if it does not go on too long. If this lack of foresight continues, however, the future of your business may be compromised, because you are probably ignoring three essential survival strategies: (1) planning the pace of business growth, (2) developing a quality assurance component, and (3) securing financial support for growth options.

PLANNING THE PACE OF GROWTH

According to Suzanne Hall Johnson, of Hall Johnson Communications, Inc., there are two main errors that entrepreneurs can make in planning for a company's growth: overextension and neglect of new product line development.

> Overextension occurs when an entrepreneur attempts to serve too many market segments at once, diffusing resources and leaving the entrepreneur exhausted. Pricing decisions can generate growth that the entrepreneur is unprepared to handle. If the entrepreneur undercharges for a service, clients may be generated, but the resulting overwork also leads to fatigue. At the other extreme is the entrepreneur who neglects to prepare for the time when a particular service is not in demand and does not have a new product line ready to go when the market changes. In order to survive, the entrepreneur must engage in balanced product line development. A useful guide is to develop one service at a time; do not add another service until that first one is going well with little attention. A reasonable approach is to spend 75 percent of your time on the current service to make sure it continues to go well and spend 25 percent of your effort on research and development in order to meet emerging market demands.

This advice can be boiled down into three basic recommendations that should form the underpinning of your survival and growth efforts.

1. As you build your company, remember to identify the pace at which you can grow without stretching your available resources.

2. Price your services at a level that gives you adequate compensation for your time and energy.

3. Integrate new product line development into your activity plans. When you have settled on a growth pattern that is appropriate for your business, you can institute the quality assurance mechanisms necessary to ensure that you achieve that growth.

MANAGING QUALITY ASSURANCE

Quality assurance is simply a control system that allows the entrepreneur to ensure that what is supposed to be happening in the business actually is happening. It is a measure of performance. An effective quality assurance system includes clearly stated outcome criteria (e.g., closer adherence to the budget, improved job performance, better patient outcomes), assigned responsibility for evaluation, and corrective action to be taken whenever there is any deviation from expected outcomes.

Many quality assurance systems generate both feedforward and feedback information (see Figure 8.1). *Feedback* information, which is obtained at the end of a process, indicates how well outcome criteria were met; *feed-forward* information, which is obtained during the process, allows you to correct any deviations to ensure that end results match established outcome standards. *Input* comprises all the information and activities that will make the system work. For example, in a staffing system, input would include the budgeted staffing, the patient acuity, and the sick and absent calls for a shift on a particular unit. *Process* refers to actions taken to measure ongoing progress toward attainment of the desired outcome(s). In the staffing example, the process might be to review all input information two hours before each shift and then to adjust staffing to meet demand. In this way, the manager can use feedforward information to take corrective action and ensure that staffing levels are acceptable levels, instead of waiting for an end-of-month budget deviation analysis to find out that staffing levels were not acceptable.

An effective quality assurance system has the following characteristics.

1. Objective outcome criteria are defined.

2. Critical points at which progress will be evaluated are identified, and corrective actions are taken when deviations are discovered.

3. Evaluation strategies fit the plans, climate, and individuals of the organization.

4. The quality assurance mechanism is flexible and economical.

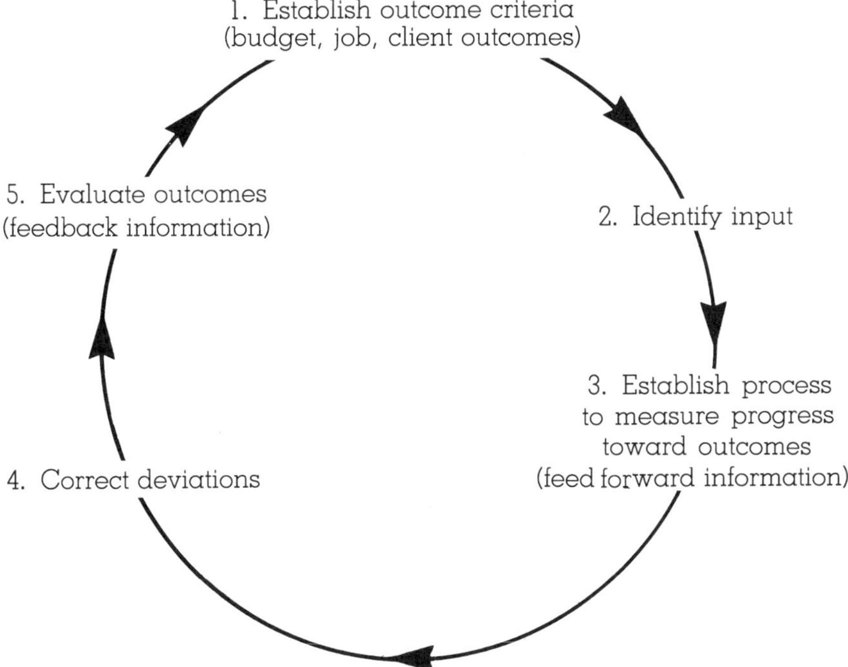

Figure 8.1 An example of a quality assurance process.

In other words, a quality assurance system should fit the business for which it is designed and provide information about progress toward goals in an efficient manner.

Most of us who worked in traditional settings before becoming nurse entrepreneurs have been involved in a quality assurance process. In fact, one facet of that process, peer review, is something that many nurses miss when they start out on their own and find that they have no one to provide collegial insight into, support for, or feedback on their ideas and actions. Without some form of quality assurance, it is difficult to predict outcomes, differentiate effective from noneffective client interventions, control a budget, or measure employee effectiveness.

Nurse entrepreneurs develop a variety of quality assurance methods, depending on the type of business they operate, their personal style, and the amount of external regulation imposed on their business. Some keep the process informal; others institute a formal program. Compare several different quality assurance strategies before selecting the one that you consider appropriate for your business.

Quality Assurance in Private Practice

Nurses in private practice have a direct link to their patients and are in a good position to monitor both the quality assurance process and the outcomes of their interventions. Karen Bonnell Wern, whose practice consists of private and group psychotherapy, mental health consultation, and education, works with adolescents and adults, primarily female. In an effort to enhance her ability to evaluate treatment effectiveness, she has recently drafted a self-report evaluation questionnaire for clients to fill out after termination of treatment.

Dr. Candice Tellis, who provides psychotherapy and wellness counseling to children and adults, relies on a few practical indicators for feedback on practice success.

> I look at my profit every three months and analyze client referral sources, etc. In private practice you function at a level of excellence—it's your livelihood, you're not dependent on an institution. You know you're giving quality if clients refer other clients and professionals keep referring; that's all you need.

Lenore Boles and Linda Hackett, of Nurse Counseling Group, include peer review in their quality assurance process.

> We have peer review one hour a week, formally structured, and spend hours on the phone weekly with each other informally. We also send a letter with nursing diagnosis and care plan to referring physicians and a follow-up letter upon termination, stating outcome.

These nurses, like many others, designed their own quality assurance systems. Often, however, nurses must adhere to specific quality assurance guidelines, either because of legislative review guidelines or because they will not be reimbursed by a third-party payer if they do not. For example, Michael Johnson, of Consulting Opinion, Inc., who develops home care and other long-term care programs with an aging emphasis, finds that "many of the programs I develop are subject to local, state and federal regulatory review." In patient care businesses, whether the focus is private practice, programmatic, or staffing related, the nurse may develop a quality assurance process that fits the business itself, but he or she may also be required to implement a formal system for reimbursement or regulatory certification. The same is true in education and consulting businesses.

Quality Assurance in Education and Consulting

Nurses providing educational programs assess both the learning process and outcomes in several ways. Dr. Eileen K. Austin, of Eileen K. Austin, Inc., offers management consultation inservice programs, continuing education, records review, and home study courses to "help agencies and individuals achieve their highest potential." She uses an "exit conference with clients to review work and a semiannual analysis of work" to evaluate service quality. Specific process indicators, such as the "reduced rate of documentation errors," are also quality indicators.

Another example of an education business is that of Dr. Carolyn Brose, of Nu-Vision, Inc., who acts as a consultant, presents workshops and seminars, and supplies computer/videodisk products. Her clients are schools of nursing and nursing organizations. Her quality assurance process includes two key elements: "I use a structured review and audit process for all courseware developed, and I gather evaluative input from all consultation, workshops, and seminars."

The experience of two nurse organizational consultants illustrates different ways in which quality review can be implemented in a business. Geneie Everett Fellows, of Humanistic Programming and Planning, evaluates the success of her interventions as a facilities consultant.

> After a facility is completed, occupied, and operational for a specified time, an evaluation is done to test planning concepts, space adequacy, functional relationships, user satisfaction, and overall planning success.

Margaret O'Brien, of Margaret Y. O'Brien—Healthcare Consultants, describes a process and outcome approach to measuring quality.

> During every project, a list of what has been done is reviewed by peers. After a project is completed, reports etc. are dissected to see what's missing, what could be better, plus what was good! Corrective actions are taken.

Maintaining the quality of a product/serevice is essential for staying in business. Besides maintaining quality, however, the nurse entrepreneur must stay tuned to the market and be ready to grow and expand at the appropriate time.

DIRECTIONS FOR SMALL BUSINESS GROWTH

There are four directions in which a small business may grow: (1) toward suppliers, (2) toward customers, (3) into related businesses, and (4) into unrelated businesses. Choosing the direction in which you will proceed involves strategic planning that is based on the strengths of your company and aimed at determining the most promising growth alternative available in your present circumstances.

Toward Suppliers

Both service and manufacturing firms purchase supplies/services from outside vendors. One way of encouraging the growth of your business is to begin in-house production of what you had been purchasing from others. Remember, however, that although in-house production can be an effective strategy, it is not a viable alternative to all outside purchasing.

To determine whether you should implement this growth strategy, take the following steps. First, identify all the supplies/services you purchase. Second, identify the supplies/services that are critical to your business; these should be considered for in-house production. Third, ask yourself these questions.

- Would such a move increase or decrease the quality of my product/service?
- Would it increase or decrease the price of my product/service?
- Would it improve or decrease availability and control of the component(s) I currently purchase from outside vendors?
- Compared with the other ways in which this business could expand, is this the best growth strategy for my business?

The answers to these questions will help you decide if growth toward your suppliers is an appropriate strategy for your business.

Toward Customers

Another growth strategy is to move into the market that is currently served by your customers. For example, if you owned a supplemental staffing business that supplied nurses to a home care agency, your decision to start your own home health care corporation would turn a former client into a competitor. The primary danger of this strategy is possible alienation of present customers. Your ability to implement this strategy depends largely on your firm's marketing skill. Before choosing this strategy option, ask yourself these questions.

- Is the reward for implementing this strategy significant?
- Does your firm (or do I) possess the marketing skill to negotiate this strategy successfully?
- What effect will this strategy have on my current business?
- Can I afford to alienate my present customers?
- Compared with the other ways in which this business could expand, is this the best growth strategy for my business?

Into Related Businesses

Business expansion through growth into related areas is one of the most popular of the growth options and a common growth choice for nurses. The experience of two nurses who responded to our questionnaire illustrates how this is accomplished.

Susan Reuler started Professional Nursing Associates, a business that provided educational services and supplemental staffing. When the demand for the staffing component increased, and other firms attempted to buy that component, she started a second business, American Nursing Resources, which was devoted to supplemental staffing. The two business cover related areas, but provide different benefits for her.

> ANR was started to fill an identified need for a nurse-run agency, by nurses and for nurses. We are the best at the business of nursing. ANR provides a secure income—there will always be a need for hospital staff nurses and private duty, hi-tech, home care nurses. PNA provides an added income and the opportunity to market myself as a nurse who has made it in business.

Adeline Laforet, of Health Care Professionals, Ltd., discovered that diversification was both a growth strategy and a survival strategy. When she started her business, in 1975, it was a supplemental staffing agency. Between 1980 and 1982, three distinct businesses emerged: staffing, certified home health care, and home care health support. In 1987, these were combined under the holding company, Health Care Professionals, Ltd.

> In 1984, after nine years of success in the staffing business, the advent of DRGs caused a sharp decline in that industry—we looked bankruptcy in the eye. Diversification was our salvation, because the home health care industry was beginning its period of rapid expansion. Today, the balance is shifting again. It is important to stay close to the market and let the market lead you into productive areas of expansion.

Expansion into related health-care areas increases your chances of success because (1) you are more likely to succeed when you do what you know best and (2) health care is an expanding industry with excellent growth potential.

If you are interested in expanding into related areas, you should make sure that your conception of related products/services is as broad as is reasonably possible, and that these related products/services would represent good utilization of your resources and provide a healthy growth option for your company. To ascertain whether this strategy is one that you should implement, ask yourself the following questions.

- Can I find new customers for what I already provide?
- Can my current customers use what I provide in some other way?
- Can I find ways in which my current customers can increase their use of what I provide?
- Are there totally new ways in which customers can use what I provide?
- Compared with the other ways in which this business could expand, is this the best growth strategy for my business?
- Does the firm possess the necessary capabilities for satisfying the need for related products/services?
- Is there a significant reward for pursuing this line of growth?

Into Unrelated Businesses

Expanding into an unrelated business is usually the last growth alternative considered. This option is often implemented by a business which is in a mature or a declining industry. Since health care is one of the projected growth markets of the future, a nurse would not be likely to find expanding into an unrelated market an attractive growth option.

MANAGING GROWTH FINANCES

Growth requires financial support, which can come from either internal or external sources. It would help you, as a new entrepreneur, to have a precise formula outlining how fast you could grow without getting into trouble; unfortunately, however, no such formula exists. The best sources of information on your optimal growth rate are internal documents that monitor the state of your business. Your most important documentation will come from your cash flow analysis and cash flow forecasts. If these documents provide accurate and reliable data, cash management is not difficult.

There is, however, one major pitfall that could nullify all your financial projections: extremely rapid growth. The rule of thumb for fast growth is that your business is in danger of outgrowing its capital structure with every increase in sales or billings on the order of 40 to 50 percent (Drucker, 1985). Furthermore, growth affects more than the capital structure of your company: it influences virtually every aspect of the business—management, staffing, systems, and controls. Therefore, whenever any one part of your plan is out of control, you must try to determine how it is affecting all the other parts of the business.

Prepare all your financial projections and forecasts for one, three, and five years. Predict your financial requirements well before the money is actually needed. With a year's lead time, you can usually obtain the necessary capital in the form that you are seeking (debt or equity investment), at a price you are willing to pay. In addition to securing the equity financing discussed in chapter 7, certain business will find it worthwhile to "go public."

Going Public

The growth and expansion of your business will require frequent and often quite large infusions of cash. One method for obtaining these infusions is to go public, that is, to sell stock in the business. Whether going public is worthwhile depends on two considerations: (1) what you will get out of the exchange (e.g., money or other benefits) and (2) whether the investor will realize sufficient benefits from his or her investing.

Benefits. From the standpoint of your company, the main legitimate reasons for going public are raising money and achieving benefits that will contribute to making your company bigger and better. The money you raise by going public may enable you to accomplish certain money-oriented tasks: (1) withdrawing some of your own investment from the company; (2) paying off existing loans; (3) expanding the company without incurring additional debt; (4) buying equipment, (5) enhancing specific sections of the business, such as marketing or research and development; or (6) setting up a mechanism that will make obtaining future financing easier. Beyond its usefulness as a money-raising tool, going public has certain prestige benefits, such as (1) increased public awareness of your firm and its products/services and (2) the ability to attract employees with more experience and credentials.

Characteristics That Appeal to Investors. There are certain characteristics that make a company an attractive investment prospect to an investor. Probably the most important of these are

- a well developed product and a good marketing capability,
- some sort of leadership in its field,
- an annual growth potential of 30 to 50 percent,
- capable management,
- current sales of $10 to 20 million, and
- a current income of about $1 million (Fritz, 1987).

You can be confident your company will be attractive to investors if it has these characteristics.

Disadvantages. There are also significant disadvantages to going public, and it is important that you recognize them and consider how they may affect you and your company. The disadvantages can be classified into two major categories: (1) loss of control (2) expense.

Loss of Control. The loss of control that an entrepreneur experiences when making a company public is the result of having brought other people into the business. As the founder of your company, you have a vision and aspirations that require a long-term or future orientation. When other people join your company as shareholders, however, they may be more interested in short-term profits than in the company's long-term interests. Such differences in viewpoint are important because shareholders are involved in your firm's decision-making processes. They are, for example, responsible for approving your board of directors, which makes decisions about how the company is run. These decisions can create more pressure on you to maintain or increase earnings, profits, and dividends. If the shareholders gain a controlling interest in the firm, you may become an employee, rather than an owner.

Another type of loss of control has to do with what information about the firm is disclosed to outsiders. You may be forced to provide information about your salary and the salary of other managers. Your company's financial state, your methods of operation, and your relationships with employees, clients, and suppliers may all be considered fair game for disclosure.

A less obvious loss of control associated with going public arises from the unpredictability of the stock market. The stock market is influenced by a tremendous number of factors that have nothing to do with your business; and these factors may cause the price of your stock to rise or fall without regard to your actual performance. A drop in the stock market means a decline in your net worth, even when business has never been better for your company.

Expense. The expense incurred in going public derives from two separate sources: (1) fees/commissions and (2) additional work that is necessary to ensure conformity with government regulations and stockholder information needs. If you are trying to raise $3 million or less, it is not uncommon to incur expenses that will absorb 20 percent of that amount.

Since only 5 percent of all US firms are publicly held, a full consideration of this topic is beyond the scope of this book (Birch, 1987). More information is available from the Securities and Exchange Commission. Write to the Office of Public Affairs, US Securities and Exchange Commission, 450 Fifth Street NW, Washington, DC 20549, for a brochure called *Q&A: Small Business and the SEC*.

In this section, we have discussed finances as they affect a company's growth potential. There is one further aspect of managing finances that you should consider: profit management. If you are not using your profits to foster the growth of the business, you should put them to work for the business in some other way—investments, for example. If you do not, your profits will become a tax liability. Since the tax laws are currently in flux, you should work closely with a financial advisor to reduce that tax liability.

Part II of this book has presented information that should help prepare you to start and run a new business. By this point, you should be ready to proceed to appendix B and develop a beginning business plan. This plan may be sufficient for your start-up needs, it may lead you to identify areas in which you require professional help, or it may act as a catalyst for the plan that ultimately guides and directs your business. This is the time to get ready, set, and grow.

III THE NURSE ENTREPRENEUR AS CONSULTANT

Because nurse entrepreneurs are perceived as innovators, experts, and role models, they are frequently approached for advice or help, even when consulting is not their primary business focus. For this reason, part III is concerned with the topic of organizational consulting. Chapter 9 presents insights into and strategies for implementing this role effectively, and chapter 10 contains an overview of the complexities of organizational consulting and reviews various methods of working through these complexities to achieve the best possible results for clients.

9 CONSULTING

Consulting is integral to the nurse entrepreneur's role. Of course, as clinical practitioners, nurses act as consultants to individuals and groups; however, many nurse entrepreneurs function in a more formalized role, that of organizational consultant. Because organizational consulting demands special expertise, this chapter is devoted to an exploration of the nature of the consulting process and the basic requirements for a successful organizational consulting practice. We examine (1) the stages of a consulting assignment, (2) the roles that nurses play in attaining the goals of a consulting assignment, (3) the skills that are essential if a nurse is to be a successful consultant, and (4) the major documents required for organization of the consulting assignment.

STAGES OF A CONSULTING ASSIGNMENT

All consulting projects are composed of five specific phases:

- entry and contracting,
- data collection and analysis,
- setting goals and planning action,
- implementation, and
- termination.

In each of these phases there are certain specific goals and tasks the achievement of which is critical for the ultimate success of the total consulting project.

Entry and Contracting

Your first contact with the client usually occurs after a series of events in the client organization: something has impelled the client to seek help.

These events may be either external or internal. The external events that can move a client to action include

- changes in the state's nurse practice act—mandating nursing diagnosis, for example;
- federal mandates, such as DRGs;
- the nursing shortage; and
- competitors' moves to increase their market share at the client's expense.

When the client organization becomes aware of these events, it must decide whether to act or to do nothing. If the client organization decides to act, it must evaluate the various action options open to it. Specifically, it must ask itself, does the urgency or importance of the situation require expertise that the organization (1) does not have, (2) could not develop in a timely manner, or (3) should not develop, since the cost (infrequent usage of the expertise, for example) of such development would be prohibitive?

The internal events that may impel a client to consider hiring a nurse consultant include

- problems with quality of nursing care that may be affecting the reputation of the institution, causing decreased physician utilization of the facility, or resulting in lawsuits;
- addition of new services/personnel (for instance, addition of the first neurosurgeon to a facility's staff, which may necessitate training the ICU nurses in neurosurgical critical care);
- inability to qualify for accreditation/endorsements from outside agencies (JCAH, for example);
- constant staff turnover or inability to recruit and retain a nurse manager for a specific unit or department, which necessitates team-building interventions;
- upgrading current services (a client may, for example, require assistance in realizing its goal of becoming a center of excellence in orthopedic nursing);
- a changeover to a different system (for instance, a move from team to primary nursing, the implementation of a career ladder, or the development of a curriculum based on a different philosophy).

Once the client has decided to retain a nurse consultant, its next step is to select the right consultant. Clients usually rely on three informational sources for referrals: (1) their own past experience with consultants, (2) recommendations made by their peers, and (3) referrals from others whom the client views as knowledgeable about consultants. These others are often power figures in the client system.

There are certain strategies that you can adopt to enhance your chances of being considered for a consulting assignment. For the client to become aware of you and your capabilities your message must be transmitted to and received by either the potential client or someone in a position to influence the potential client. Accordingly, your first step is to decide what it is you offer and to articulate this clearly in client-centered terms. Your second step is to decide how you will disseminate your message. You will be better equipped to make this decision if you have carefully targeted your customer base. There is a wide range of standard marketing methods you can use to get the word out about your services—mailing out press releases, buying advertising space, publishing books or articles, making presentations at organizations to which your client base belongs, sending letters or newsletters, hosting receptions, and so on. Use any of these strategies that might work for you, but do not limit yourself to them. There are other approaches that are just as effective, such as networking.

Networking is a powerful strategy that is highly effective in getting the word out about your business but is too often overlooked. Networking should not be limited to people you regard as especially powerful and influencial. Instead, it should extend to everyone you know—family, friends, acquaintances in professional associations, business associates, past co-workers, current customers, and other consultants. Some of these people also make up your potential client's circle of contacts, and some may be power figures in that client system.

Once the client organization has been made aware of you and your services, it may make an initial overture, which is usually to ask you to submit a proposal describing how you would approach the problem and achieve the desired results. Alternatively, the client may schedule a time at which you and a representative of the organization can sit down and discuss the problem face to face. Ultimately, either of these approaches may result in entry into the contracting engagement.

The entry and contracting phase allows both the client and the consultant to learn something about the other party and establish the basis of a working relationship. Each party is refining and defining the scope of the engagement and the nature of the proposed relationship. The consultant becomes familiar with the client organization, its resources, the people of key significance to the consulting project, and the organization's readiness for change. Each party listens to the other's expectations, agendas, and values.

If during the initial contact it becomes obvious that the client's problem requires expertise that you cannot provide, you should decline to enter into the relationship. You should also decline if the needed intervention has little or no likelihood of succeeding or if the client has hidden agendas, as in the following examples.

1. You, an inexperienced consultant, are being brought in by the board of directors or the hospital administrator to resolve a problem in the nursing department over the strenuous objections of the nursing administrator. (You could consider this assignment once you are an experienced consultant.)
2. You are being hired to spy on the nursing staff.
3. You are expected to implement a predetermined plan while making the plan seem objective to those who are being manipulated.

If, however, you are satisfied that you and the client share similar standards and values and will be able to work together, you can think about negotiating a written contract. (This will be covered in more detail later.)

Data Collection and Analysis

Now that you and your client have agreed to work together to resolve a particular problem, you will need a clearer, more comprehensive picture of the nature of that problem. In the data collection and analysis phase, you begin to bring the problem into focus. Your data collection methods will vary according to what information you decide is necessary to understand the problem in any particular case. Any of a number of approaches can be used:

- interviews;
- questionnaires;
- tests;
- studies;
- focus groups;
- direct observation;
- assessment, interpretation, and analysis of resources, documents, and standards; or
- estimation of the client's capacity for insight into the problem and inherent problem-solving ability.

When you have collected the data you need, you must analyze it. Look first for the factors that can affect—either positively or negatively—your ability to resolve the problem. Next, examine your data to ascertain whether they support the original view of the problem and the initial project goals. It often happens that a symptom of a problem is mistaken for the problem itself. A patient with a headache, for example, may fear that he has a brain tumor when the problem is actually hypertension.

Mistaking a symptom for the underlying problem is an error that consultants encounter frequently. For example, one of Advanced Health Care Concepts' clients identified its problem in what seemed clear and sensible terms: "Our nurses don't know how to do nursing diagnosis." A sample nursing diagnosis was supplied to support that contention: "Pain and knowledge deficit related to labor, delivery, and postpartum experience." Clearly, this diagnosis was unacceptably broad, but during the data collection process it became apparent that there was more to the problem than a simple knowledge deficit. The nurses were writing all-inclusive diagnoses for three reasons: first, because they were required to have a nursing diagnosis before they could chart *anything*—even the implementation of a medical order such as a bolus of LIDOCAINE for a cardiac arrhythmia required a nursing diagnosis; second, incidental narrative notes were not permitted for any reason; and third, flow sheets for routine care were not part of the hospital's system.

Under these circumstances, formulating an extremely broad diagnosis was actually quite logical: it kept the nurses from spending an inordinate amount of time on paperwork while enabling them to conform to the letter of the institution's rules. Thus, the real problem in this institution was the way in which nursing diagnosis was conceived and used, but the institution had failed to recognize this. If the project had been carried out according to the client's initial perception of the problem, it should have been doomed to failure—the nurses would still be writing extremely general, virtually useless nursing diagnoses.

When your findings conflict with the original premise of the problem, you must go back to the client to redefine and clarify the problem and the project. When that is accomplished, or when you have determined that the original conception of the problem was in fact accurate, you can move on to the next phase of the consulting process.

Setting Goals and Planning Action

In this, the goal setting and action planning phase, you must specify the goals of your intervention and the methods you will use to ensure that these goals will be achieved. Establish a logical, step-by-step approach to goal achievement that leaves nothing to chance. Be sure that your client has a clear understanding of what you require from it. Specify who will perform what activities, when, why, and how, and identify the contribution that each step of your strategy will make to the final achievement of the project's goals.

Implementation

The consultant's role in the implementation phase depends on what has been specified in the action plan. In some cases the consultant will have the sole responsibility for implementation, whereas in others, the client may have the sole responsibility for implementation, and the consultant's job may be over when the implementation phase begins. Alternatively, the nurse consultant may act as a coordinator, facilitator, and evaluator to help the client through the implementation phase; this is more usual. Typically, the consultant's role in this phase is to ensure that the client maintains momentum and continues to progress toward accomplishment of the specified goals. Usual duties would include

- ensuring that the proper sequence of the action plan is maintained,
- teaching the client the skills needed for successful implementation,
- providing feedback to the client on the state of the project,
- keeping the client motivated to progress toward goal achievement,
- removing obstacles encountered in implementation,
- revising the action plan for improved results, and
- evaluating ongoing progress toward attainment of goals.

By the end of this phase, it may seem that the project is finished. There remains, however, one more phase: termination.

Termination

The termination phase serves several important functions. It is in this part of the assignment that the client and consultant review what has been accomplished, what remains to be accomplished, and what is required for follow-up or continued support. In particular, the consultant is looking for indications that the client knows how to retain what has been accomplished and has a clear idea of how to continue alone toward attainment of the project's remaining goals.

NURSE CONSULTANT ROLES

As you work through the stages of the consulting assignment, you may have to take on one or more different roles. Because the essential characteristics of these roles are often reminiscent of the functional characteristics associated with various occupations, the names of these occupations are sometimes used as labels for the roles. The roles most commonly assumed by nurse consultants can be labeled as follows:

- detective,
- diagnostician,
- informational expert, and
- co-contributor.

Detective

In the detective role, you will be expected to diagnose the client's problem. This role requires strong investigative skills. You must be able to determine the kind of information needed to uncover the problem, and you must be able to discern relationships between seemingly unrelated data.

Diagnostician

The diagnostician role closely reflects the medical model. In this role, the consultant is expected to diagnose the problem and prescribe the cure, and the client is expected to follow the advice and be cured of the problem. The diagnostician needs not only strong investigative skills but also the ability to prescribe measures that will overcome the client's problem. The diagnostician's role ends with the prescription: the client implements the prescribed resolution.

Informational Expert

The informational expert role actually comprises two roles: that of scientist/researcher and that of teacher.

In the scientist/researcher role, the consultant uses the scientific method to develop the project's outcome criteria and strategies and to analyze and synthesize the data. This is done according to a step-by-step procedure, which is adhered to strictly. In the scientist/researcher role, the consultant must be able to reflect on the problem in an objective manner. This role is especially useful for discovering and handling obstacles to the achievement of project goals.

In the teacher role, the consultant works to inculcate in the client those skills that will help the client to assume an active role in problem solving. It is not enough that the consultant knows how to solve the problem: he or she must be able to impart that knowledge to the client. The teacher role is most likely to be appropriate when the client and consultant decide to work collaboratively or when the client will be assuming responsibility for the implementation phase.

Co-contributor

In the co-contributor role, the consultant and client work collaboratively to achieve the goals of the project. To fulfill this role successfully, the consultant must have excellent communication and coordination skills and be able to work with the client as a partner, not as a boss or an underling.

Benefits of Identifying Role

Being able to label the role you are playing at any point in your consulting assignment yields several benefits.

- It gives you a quick reference point that helps you to organize your approach.
- It provides a framework for each portion of the project.
- It adds to your knowledge of which roles are appropriate or inappropriate for which situations.
- It helps you to determine which specific duties you will perform.
- It ensures that the interventions you implement are suitable to the role you have assumed.

Factors Affecting Consultant's Choice of Roles

Which roles you assume in the course of your consulting depends on (1) your personal beliefs, strengths, and limitations; (2) your experience; (3) the client's expectations; (4) how well your norms and standards match the client's; and (5) various unrelated events that affect the consulting project.

The personal beliefs, strengths, and limitations that you bring to an assignment color virtually every aspect of that assignment. For example, if you believe that the client's goals are most likely to be achieved when the client acquires ownership of the problem and commits itself to the methods that must be applied to resolve the problem, you will probably choose the co-contributor role to handle the parts of the assignment associated with those tasks.

Your experience is inevitably a factor as well. When you encounter problems that are similar or identical to some that you have already encountered, you will naturally assume roles that have worked before and avoid those that have not.

The client's expectations—which reflect the *client's* experiences, beliefs, strengths, and limitations—also influence your role choices. For example, if the client has exhausted its diagnostic capabilities without being able to determine what the problem is, the client may expect the consultant to assume the role of diagnostician.

The extent to which your norms and standards match those of your client always influences your selection of roles. The greater the differences between your norms and standards and your client's, the more you will need to assume a role that gives you maximum control over the project. If the differences are few or insignificant, you will probably choose a role like that of informational expert, in which you help the client to develop skills that will enable it to assume more responsibility for the implementation phase of the project.

The potential effect of unrelated events on the consulting project should not be underestimated. Whenever unrelated events create a change in the client institution or in the outlook of the project, your roles may change. One example of an unrelated event that might affect your choice of role would be a hospital's decision to replace all its nursing service administrators in the middle of a project. Another would be a hospital administration's decision to cut institutional expenses by no longer paying nurses to attend in-house educational programs.

Recently, Nancy Doleysh, of Advanced Health Care Concepts, faced precisely the situation outlined by the second example. The decision had been made without any consideration of the impact that the policy change would have on the educational component of a consulting project to prepare ICU nurses for expanded duties and the utilization of technologies new to the institution. This policy change was of grave concern to the consultant, because its implementation would have meant the waste of tremendous amount of money that the client had committed to the project, and because failure to achieve a project's goals often has a negative effect on a consultant's reputation. The consultant assumed the detective role in an effort to ascertain the precise monetary and other implications that implementation of this policy change would have on the client organization. When the client was confronted with this information, it was deciding, after some consideration, to abandon the policy change and implement a cost-cutting alternative that would save money without interfering with the achievement of the project's goals and the concomitant return on the client's investment.

SKILLS OF THE SUCCESSFUL CONSULTANT

The skills associated with success as a consultant fall under three headings: (1) those that are important for running the business, (2) those that are important for carrying out the mechanical aspects of the consulting project, and (3) those that are important for motivating the client to enter into the project and implement the consultant's recommendations. At this point, you will find it helpful to refer back to the assessments in chapter 2. The business and entrepreneurial skills described there are as applicable to a consulting practice as they are to any other enterprise.

Throughout all the phases of a consulting project, success depends on the consultant's skills and abilities in the following areas:

- professional nursing,
- communication,
- problem solving,
- conflict management,
- interpersonal relationships,
- diagnostic capabilities,
- self-confidence,
- honesty,
- keen insight into people and situations,
- logical thinking,
- flexibility,
- creativity,
- innovation,
- ability to cope with rejection,
- strong grounding in the theory relevant to a consulting practice,
- patience, and
- ability to tolerate ambiguity.

The ability to motivate a client to enter into a consulting relationship, talk frankly about a problem, or implement the recommendations you make requires a unique blend of skills. To motivate clients effectively you must implement your skills strategically, even therapeutically, as client need dictates. The method you use to do this bears a striking resemblance to the nursing process. Client motivation is enhanced when the client sees you as

- perceptive and sensitive to the feelings and needs of others,
- genuinely interested in helping,

- supportive of the client's efforts to change,
- ethical,
- nonjudgmental,
- empathetic,
- articulate,
- persuasive,
- confidence inspiring,
- sincere,
- trustworthy,
- optimistic,
- charismatic,
- competent,
- credible,
- consistent, and
- decisive

Because organizational consulting offers the opportunity to use a wide range of skills, most consultants find this occupation challenging and exciting. The satisfaction you feel when you have helped an organization "turn itself around" is exhilarating. Our goal in this review of the consulting process has been to help you find that feeling of satisfaction in your own consulting work. In the final section of the chapter, we review the documentation component of a consulting practice, since this is the component that gives your consulting activity its legal status.

DOCUMENTS THAT ORGANIZE A CONSULTING PRACTICE

Proposals and contracts with clients and individuals with whom you subcontract are essential consulting documents. Accordingly, the following section focuses on presenting information that will enhance your ability either to develop your own documents or to make use of the expertise of an attorney or other professional advisors, when necessary.

Requests for Proposals

When clients have a need whose solution requires outside expertise, they may tender a request for a proposal. This is their way of letting you know that they are interested in what you can do, how you would help them with their problem, and how much your assistance would cost. By responding to a request for a proposal, you enable the client to determine how applicable your expertise is to their problems.

The client's request for a proposal generally includes instructions that help you provide the desired information. Each project is unique and generates different requirements; consequently, your proposal's structure can range from extremely simple to highly complex, depending on the specific requirements of the project. A simple proposal would include at least five parts:

- a description of the work to be done,
- the name of the individual who will perform the work,
- a description of the services or personnel to be supplied by the client,
- the amount of time that the project will take and when you will begin work, and
- a description of the types and amounts of fees to be paid by the client and the dates the fees are due.

Standard Proposal

The body of a standard proposal is usually made up of four sections.

1. *Introduction*. The introduction tells who you are and summarizes your qualifications. The second summary in the introduction describes the client's problem and needs. Your understanding of the client's needs may derive from information implied or stated in initial communications, from the request for a proposal, from telephone conversations, or from meetings with the client.
2. *Discussion*. The discussion provides an in-depth description of the client's problem and the measures you would implement to correct it. An additional objective is to demonstrate that you have the expertise, creativity, and capabilities necessary to resolve the problem.
3. *Proposed program*. This section includes a more in-depth exploration of the program you would use to address the client's problem. Typically, you list the project's objectives, organizational features, and benefits; describe the persons who will be involved in accomplishing the objectives of the project, the quality assurance methodology, the time schedules, and end results of the project; and add other documentation, such as resumes and charts, as needed.

4. *Experience and qualifications*. In this section, you verify that you have the ability and experience to do the required work in a dependable, professional manner. You may wish to include a list of articles or books you have written about the area in which you are consulting, a description of the variety and extent of professional experience you possess and any relevant special education/degrees you have, or a mention of any recognition (as a speaker, for example), awards, or honors you have earned in the present consulting area. If you have had assignments of this type before and know that your former clients will provide good references, you may wish to include their names in this section.

An example of a standard proposal for one of Advanced Health Care Concepts' consulting assignments is provided in appendix C. In this particular proposal, a description of the company, the names of the consultants, and a list of professional references were included in the cover letter. Additional supporting documentation included a class outline, a class schedule, and objectives for a specific class.

Formal Proposal

In some circumstances, a formal proposal may be appropriate. Such a proposal contains numerous sections that explain virtually every aspect of your proposed program. It usually includes the following 18 components (Gray, 1985).

1. *Table of Contents*.
2. *Introduction*. In this section, you demonstrate the client's need. State that the need is important, requires professional intervention, is of interest to you, and can best be influenced by your expertise.
3. *Project purpose*. State the purpose and goals of the project in the client's own words; this helps the client identify with your proposal. By making goals measurable, you assure the client that progression towards those goals will be apparent.
4. *Project benefits*. Here you define the benefits the client will derive from hiring your firm for this project.
5. *Approach, scope, and plan*. If several approaches to the client's problem are feasible, you should mention all of them. Explain which of the various possible approaches you will take and why. Establish a time frame for the project, and break large tasks down into smaller ones, so that the client can more easily determine

whether the project is progressing according to plan. Be sure to provide enough information to allow the client to decide if your plan seems reasonable and your expertise appropriate. Consider how much and what type of information you need to provide to achieve that objective; do not offer too much. If you tell the client organization too much about the processes and techniques you will use in the project, it may be able to complete the project without you.

6. *Project schedule*. List the activities that must be performed and the order in which they will be performed.

7. *Progress reports*. Communication between you and your client increases the confidence your client has in you, improves your chances of getting paid, and reduces the likelihood that serious misunderstandings will arise and jeopardize the project. Specify the intervals at which you will submit progress reports to ensure that communication will be maintained.

8. *Costing summary*. Your client will want to know how you bill your time, what your billing procedures are, and how you handle those expenses that the client is expected to pay.

9. *Personnel and qualifications*. Briefly describe the history of your firm and the qualifications of your consulting personnel. If you have solved similar problems in the past, say so.

10. *Subcontracts*. State which portions of the project will be subcontracted and to whom they will be subcontracted. If the client will be bearing some of the responsibility for the technical performance of the subcontracted personnel, you must specify the nature and extent of the responsibility.

11. *Use of client personnel*. If the fee you have quoted is contingent on utilization of the client's personnel, be sure to spell out which and how many people you will need, what duties they will perform, and how long they will be needed.

12. *Senior management support*. In this section, you acknowledge that the support of senior management members throughout the institution is vital to the success of the project. Specify the purpose and frequency of the meetings that will involve these senior managers.

13. *Steering committee function*. Members of the institution's staff may be assigned to provide for implementation of the consultant's work. If such a committee is to be formed, you should detail its composition, duties, and responsibilities here.

14. *Output material included.* In this section, list any products that are part of the project, such as videotapes, class outlines, reports, and assessments.

15. *Management plan.* A contact person within the organization will be delegated to assist with questions or problems that arise in the implementation of the project. Identify that person and describe his or her duties and authority in regard to the project.

16. *Disclaimers.* Consultants are retained in an advisory capacity and have no real authority; thus, even if a consultant gives excellent advice, a project may fail to achieve its objectives if the client rejects this advice. Disclaimers reiterate this point and outline the consultant's responsibilities and options if his or her recommendations are not followed. In addition, they establish ownership and control of proprietary information, such as videotapes or other instructional materials.

17. *References.* The opinion of former clients may influence a prospective client to choose you for a particular project. When using former clients as references, you should obtain their written permission to do so, and you should make contact with them to verify that they do indeed continue to think highly of you and the work you did for them.

18. *Summary and closing of proposal.* In this final section, you attempt to move the client to act and to choose you as the consultant best equipped to handle the assignment. Express your belief in the necessity of the project, make yourself available to answer questions, and indicate that you are prepared to begin work as soon as the client makes the decision to carry out the project.

An additional advantage of writing a formal proposal for a client's project is that the proposal can later be used as the contract between the parties or as the basis for the contract.

Contracts

The question that is most often asked about contracts is, "Do I need them?" There are persuasive arguments on both sides of the question, as consultation of the sources will show. To decide whether a contract is necessary in your situation, examine the advantages and disadvantages outlined below.

Advantages. A major advantage of a contract is that it protects both parties against misunderstandings. Defining all aspects of the agreement makes everyone concerned aware of his or her duties, rights, and responsibilities. In addition, it gives you a professional image, protects you from an untruthful client, secures your interests in the event of the death or discharge of the individual with whom you made the agreement, prevents a project from being extended without renegotiation of the fee, and may serve as collateral for financing your company.

Disadvantages. A major disadvantage of a written contract is that it may make a client uncomfortable. If you insist upon a contract as a condition of doing business, the client may feel that your intentions are less than honorable and may be reluctant to do business. To ensure that its interests are adequately represented, the client may incur additional expenses by having an attorney peruse the document. A contract may not be worthwhile for projects involving small amounts of money, since the additional costs incurred may double the total price of the project.

If the disadvantages of a written contract seem to outweigh the advantages, there is an alternative you should consider: a letter of intent. The letter of intent comprises a general description of the work to be done, a determination of the amount to be paid, and a waiver documenting that either party may terminate the agreement on sufficient prior notice (the length of which should be specified). The letter of intent is signed by you and by a responsible executive of the client organization. It may be used in lieu of a standard contract (see appendix D).

Formal Contracts. The structure of the formal contract varies according to the situation. The example in appendix E contains

- the names of the parties involved,
- the terms of the contract,
- the duties of the consultant,
- the duties of the client,
- the payment of fees schedule,
- a description of how consultant expenses are to be handled,
- a statement that the written agreement represents the sum total of the entire agreement, and
- the signatures of the contracting parties.

This contract was developed from information sent to the client in response to their request for a proposal. The agreement between the client and the consultant did in fact cover such points as permission for the consultant to use the institution's name in advertising, utilization of subcontractors for portions of the work, reassurance that the client's problems would remain confidential, and establishment of ownership of all videotapes, outlines, policies, and procedures produced during the course of the project. If verbal agreement on these matters had been deemed inadequate, these points would have been addressed in the written contract.

Other elements that might be required in a contract include

- specification of what happens when fees are not paid within prearranged time. A typical approach to avoiding late fees is to charge interest at a rate higher than that charged by banks.
- a clause that describes the conditions under which the consultant will stop providing services, such as failure of the client to pay the consultant.
- a statement that the consultant is an independent contractor and is therefore exempt from the client's tax withholding obligations.
- a description of the services that will be subcontracted.
- a statement that the consultant will regard information about the client organization as confidential.
- a description of the ownership of materials or ideas resulting from the consultant's services.
- permission to use the client's name for advertising purposes.
- a description of the process to be used to resolve disagreements between the contracting parties.
- a description of the conditions of termination. Usually either party is permitted to terminate the relationship by giving notice of a prescribed number of days.

The contract in appendix E contains components that might logically go into continuing education subcontracts. They are:

- Program. This section identifies the specific project for which the subcontractor is being retained.
- Identification of subcontractor. This section includes pertinent information for several purposes. The line with "Name" on it also is used to list the social security number, since that information is required on 1099 forms, which are filed at the end of the year. Information about qualifications is used in introducing the speaker

at the program, and it is also used as supporting documentation when requesting ANA recognition for the program's continuing education units.

- Details of the program. The individual's job description—coordinator, instructor—is included here, as well as the description of where and when the program will be presented.
- Compensation. The money value of the contract, as well as conditions under which the contract is invalid.
- Signatures of both the contractor and contractee are included, along with the date the document was signed.
- Audiovisual equipment requests on the contract form obviates the need for another form or separate correspondence.
- Teaching materials deadlines ensure that there will be sufficient time to type or copy materials for distribution.

Management of paperwork can be a frustrating battle that consumes enormous amounts of time and energy. Since most entrepreneurs are action-oriented, they tend to feel trapped in the "paper jungle." If you make the effort to understand what documentation is essential for your business purposes and to set up a system for managing it as effortlessly as possible, you can reduce the stress you are under to a minimum.

The process described in this chapter is one that is used by most consultants. Nurse entrepreneurs, however, bring to their consulting activities a unique vision that increases their value to the organizations fortunate enough to retain their services. In chapter 10, we explore strategies for integrating that nursing vision into your consulting practice.

10 THE NURSE AS ORGANIZATIONAL CONSULTANT

Organizations are complex dynamic systems that test the consultant's skills. Nurses bring unique strengths to the role of organizational consultant: namely, their understanding of patients and nurses (the organization's major assets) and their experience with a holistic approach to diagnosis and intervention. These strengths enhance nurses' ability to ascertain how effectively an organization's subsystems support nursing and patient care outcomes. A nurse's vision of a healthy health care organization would be one in which the goals of nurses, patients, and the corporation are necessarily congruent. Nurses make a difference organizationally because they integrate nursing concepts at three critical points in the consultation: (1) organizational analysis, (2) the change process, and (3) assessment of the organizational culture.

ORGANIZATIONAL ANALYSIS

Nurses are experienced at assessing a whole system through analysis of its interrelated subsystems. Dr. Vicki Lachman, RN, PhD, of V L Associates, explains the benefits of her systems approach to consulting in her brochure:

> Dr. Lachman's expertise in diagnosing the core organizational system and management problems and then designing creative solutions has gained her a reputation as a fine detective and teacher.

The positive reputation that nurse consultants like Dr. Lachman develop springs from that integration of nursing and organizational concepts for the purpose of analyzing and restructuring the dynamics occurring at various levels of an organization. Complex organizations are best analysed with the aid of a structured process that focuses attention on all the major components of the organization and permits systematic review of the data collected.

Organizational Components

Frame and associates (1982) identify six organizational components that must be analyzed prior to any change effort:

1. groups, which can be analyzed according to norms, relationships (both within and between groups), performance levels, work distribution, functions, priorities, and decision-making and problem-solving processes;
2. environment, which is established by the market, competitors, related organizations, government regulations, societal values, manpower potential, and social responsiveness;
3. technology, which consists of knowledge, equipment, processes used, and the overall flow of activity;
4. structure, which includes the reward system, the hierarchy, patterns of contact between employees, the goals and purposes of the organization, policies and procedures, the financial system, the physical setting, decision making mechanisms, size, and reporting relations;
5. individuals, who possess unique biographies, skills, educational backgrounds, needs, motivational patterns, value systems, behavior patterns, and performance levels; and
6. tasks, which reflect job-design elements, authority and responsibility, necessary skills, time requirements, motivational patterns, and work flow.

A client's problems arise from one or more of these components. The six components are so closely interrelated that even when you are implementing a change process that directly involves only one or two of them, you must still take pains to assess the impact of the change on all the other components. You must evaluate the data obtained from analysis of each of these areas to determine how it fits into the subsystems of the organization, so that you can identify appropriate targets for change.

Organizational Subsystems

Organizations are comprised of three subsystems that contribute equally to the success of their endeavors: (1) the sociosystems, (2) the process system, and (3) the technosystem. The sociosystem consists of the attitudes, values, and perceptions of the employees coupled with the climate in the organization, which is a function of the degree of openness, trust, cooperation, and self-direction present. The process system consists of the organization's decision-making, communication, and problem-solving vehicles, which incorporate such elements as problem definition, selection of solutions, utilization of resources, delegation of tasks, conflict management, goal setting, information sharing, and self-evaluation. The technosystem consists of the organization's technical and structural aspects: formalized procedures, policies, and rules, as well as the design of the organization, staffing patterns, physical facilities, equipment, tools, and operating technology (Frame, Hess, & Nielsen, 1982).

This subsystem classification provides an instructive and useful conceptual framework that helps you to evaluate problem areas and formulate resolutions that address a specific subsystem's problems while maintaining a balance between the three subsystems. The case study that follows illustrates how this framework can be used to analyze the problems of a department within an organization.

Case Study: Integrating Staff Development

This case study is developed from several consulting projects and does not represent one specific organization.

History. A small health-care facility had remained stable for several years, with few additions in services or increases in patient population. Many employees were "old-timers," and the overall climate was one of the "family." Conflicts were usually smoothed over, and employees tended to be protected rather than required to improve their performance. The institution was a centralized but not a highly formalized one; there were few structured meetings, and only essential policies, procedures, and guideline were spelled out and enforced.

Within a two-year period, however, the organization responded dramatically to the economic pressures being felt in the health-care environment. Several new services were added, and plans were made to add others in the near future. The organization was decentralized, except for certain functions, such as quality assurance and education. New staff members were recruited and added rapidly. Productivity and cost containment were increasingly emphasized, and managers' roles changed as their authority and responsibility for product line management increased. The department most affected by these changes was the nursing department. The newly hired nurse administrator requested consulting assistance because of increasing conflicts surrounding the staff development function, which remained centralized. After a period of analysis, the consultant was able to identify the problems using a subsystem framework. The problems are listed in Table 10.1.

Consequences of Problems. The overall result of these problems is that a collaborative process for utilizing staff development is difficult to implement. New staff members start employment on dates determined by the managers and there is no coordination for orientation. Staff members in the critical care areas are complaining about inadequate orientation, and turnover in these areas has increased. There is no cohesive philosophy of staff

TABLE 10.1 Examples of Problems Discovered by Nurse Consultants in the Three Organizational Subsystems

Sociosystem	Technosystem	Process System
1. A shared philosophy that expresses the group's values, attitudes, and perceptions about staff development has not been developed.	1. The changes and growth that have occurred create different needs for and have raised questions about: • the purpose and outcomes for staff development, and • the appropriate structure for staff development (centralized versus decentralized).	1. Decision rules based on standards and criteria for learning effectiveness and organizational effectiveness are not used consistently by the whole group to make decisions about staff development or to evaluate its effectiveness.
2. Mutual accountabilities that individuals interdependent in the staff development process have toward each other are not clearly identified.	2. There are varied perceptions and a lack of clarity about the staff development coordinator role.	2. The rapid changes have demanded a high degree of flexibility from staff development, but a collaborative planning process for use of the staff development function by several decentralized units has not been established.
3. Trust and conflict issues that are part of the group's history make collaboration difficult.	3. Staff development policies and procedures do not provide structure and authority for decision making related to the function.	

continued

TABLE 10.1 (cont.)

Sociosystem	Technosystem	Process System
	4. Control mechanisms to provide the administrator with feedback about implementation of the staff development function are not in place. 5. Criteria for the administrator's intervention when the process is not adequately implemented have not been discussed and established.	3. The expectations for how and by whom problem identification, problem solving, and conflict management are to be handled are unclear and clouded by power and territory issues. 4. A mechanism for role support, decision support, and intervention when conflicts arise is lacking. 5. A formalized communication process that facilitates effective discussion of goals and problems as well as support for decision making and follow-through accountability is not in place. 6. Decentralized decisions to use a centralized function creates a fragmented rather than a cooperative departmental approach.

development. People and money resources are wasted, and productivity is impaired when staff do not receive the full benefit of a staff development effort. In a decentralized operation with centralized staff development, collaboration is essential for effective use of a scarce resource by multiple and separate clients.

In this case study, there are problems in each subsystem, and interventions must be made in each of the three interdependent subsystems simultaneously. For example, if the technosystem is altered by decentralization of staff development, changes must be made in the other two systems in order to support and reinforce that alteration. Different types of skills are required for operation within each subsystem: planning, organizing, and problem-solving skills are necessary for working within the technosystem and the process system, whereas group process skills are essential for addressing issues arising in the sociosystem. Although, the case study was concerned with subsystems in a single department, the same framework can be applied to an entire organization or used to evaluate the nursing subsystem and its relationships with other organizational subsystems.

Status of Nursing Analysis

To obtain information on the relationships between nursing and the other subsystems within an organization and determine the degree to which nursing practice is supported or blocked, ask the following questions.

Sociosystem. Here your aim is to uncover the prevalent organizational attitudes, values, and beliefs about nursing held by nurses and others within the organization.

1. Which professional nursing behaviors are valued by various groups within the organization? Specify the groups (e.g., nurses, physicians, administrators, patients).
2. Which behaviors are rejected by or evoke a negative response from various groups within the organization?
3. What happens when nurses attempt to be more self-directive in their practice? Which specific groups support that behavior, and which groups do not?
4. Are nurses' decisions about patients respected or rejected?
5. What value is placed on education for nurses?
6. How do nurses feel about themselves in this organization?
7. What is the level of role satisfaction for nurses in this organization?

Process System. Here the goal is to ascertain how well nursing is integrated into the various layers of the organization.

1. Do nurses play an active role in the identification and solution of problems related to patient care?
2. Do nurses have the opportunity to interact with other groups within the organization? Do they take advantage of these opportunities? Do they demonstrate the ability to use power and influence assertively in their intergroup communications?
3. Are nurses involved in the committee structure at all levels of the organization?
4. Are nurses able to address the conflicts they experience in an assertive way? Do they have organizational support when they do this?
5. Does the nursing philosophy that staff nurses share agree with the organizational philosophy?
6. Do the nurses' goals for patients agree with the organization's goals?
7. Are nurses utilized appropriately as a professional resource?
8. Do nurses have control over decisions related to nursing practice?

Technosystem. Here the objective is to determine the extent to which the organization's structure supports nursing.

1. Are policies, procedures, and rules sufficiently flexible to support nurses' professional decision making, or are the nurses hampered by them?
2. Do the policies, procedures, and rules appropriately reinforce and reward professional nursing practice?
3. Does the formal organizational structure recognize nursing to the same degree as it does other disciplines? (That is, are nurse managers at the same level as other managers in the organization with a similar span of control?)
4. Do nurses have easy access to the supplies and equipment they need to provide patient care?
5. Are staffing patterns based on patient's need for professional care?
6. Do nurses have access to necessary space, education, breaks, and so forth?
7. Are patient care areas designed to facilitate efficient care?

8. Do nurses receive sufficient educational support (orientation, staff development, and so forth) to prepare them for the role complexities and technologic complexities of the job?

9. Are there avenues for professional advancement for nurses who develop their expertise as caregivers, or do these nurses face the career plateau trap in this institution?

The answers to these 24 questions give a clear picture of the status of nursing in a given organization. When each answer is followed by two other questions—how does this situation create a benefit or loss to patients? and how does this help or hinder the organization?—the interdependence among nursing, patient welfare, and organizational success becomes apparent. Using the information gained in this way, the nurse consultant induces changes in each of the subsystems in order to close the gaps between desirable nursing, patient, and organizational outcomes. Those changes make a difference for nursing, as well as for patients and for the client organization.

ORGANIZATIONAL CHANGE PROCESS

Change is an alteration in the internal or external environment that necessitates a subsequent behavior alteration in an individual, group, or system. It is a staple of your work as a consultant, and it offers a considerable challenge to both you and your client. To be a successful consultant, you must have an awareness of how change affects each element of an organization and an understanding of what the sources of resistance are and how to deal with them. A consulting intervention relies on planned innovation: an orderly sequence of goal setting, planning, and systematic action designed to maximize the opportunities for success.

Change Roles

There are four roles people in an organization may assume in a situation in which change must be implemented:

1. change sponsor—the individual or group with the organizational power to legitimize change;

2. change target—the individual or group who as a result of the change will alter aspect of their skill, knowledge, attitude, or behavior

3. change advocate—individuals or groups who want change but lack sufficient sponsorship (Connor, 1985); and

4. change agent—the individual who employs his or her knowledge and skill to initiate, implement, or facilitate change in a target group.

When attempting to introduce a change effort, you may perform one or more tasks—for instance, appropriately influence sponsors, recruit advocates, or act as the change agent assisting the target group with the change process. The change process comprises the following six stages (see Figure 10.1).

Awareness/Need. Without an awareness of a need for change, the client cannot make a commitment to the change effort. Dissatisfaction with the present, a perceived gap between actual and desired results, or a discomfort with current knowledge or skill levels can be the basis for a desire for change. As a consultant, you are a catalyst that helps people recognize a need for innovation.

Planning/Goal Setting. During this stage, strategies to resolve identified problems are selected. You can enhance the planning effort by presenting a wide range of options; encouraging creative problem solving; ensuring that realistic, achievable goals and timetables are set; identifying organizational resources; and helping to establish effective control mechanisms.

Action. As a consultant, you may act in several ways to facilitate implementation of change: teaching new knowledge and skills; mobilizing resources to support the change effort; coordinating all aspects of the change

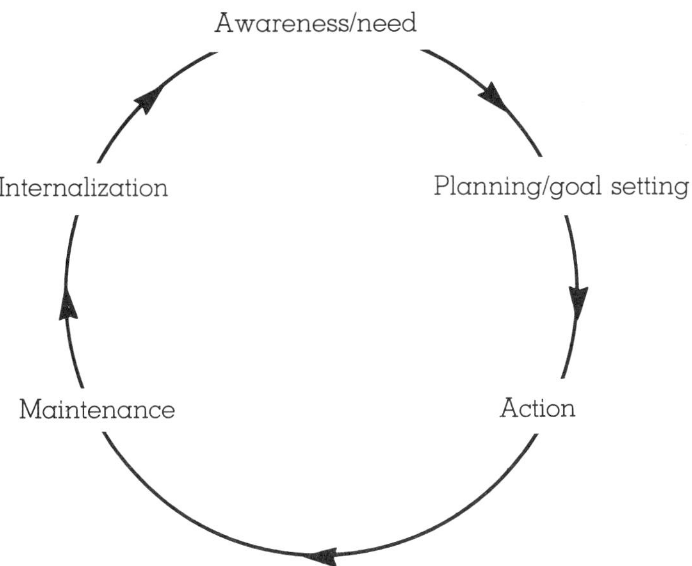

Figure 10.1 Stages of the change process.

process; and providing feedback, advice, and support, among others. In this stage, new strategies are tested, new problems are discovered, obstacles are overcome, and targeted goals are reached. Be sure to monitor all interrelated organizational systems and confirm their continuing support for the change.

Maintenance. This stage is often neglected. It often happens that once the change appears to be operative, all the support mobilized for the initial implementation is withdrawn, under the assumption that the change has been accomplished. At this point, staff members may still feel uncertain about their new skills, or they may begin to discover new problems related to the change, and the temptation to revert to "the good old days" may be too strong to resist. Your job in this stage is to maintain the momentum of the change by providing feedback that recognizes growth, assisting with problem resolution, and pacing the withdrawal of support resources in accordance with the observable increases in staff competence. When a pattern of consistent use of new behaviors emerges, commitment to the change has been internalized.

Internalization. When new concepts and behaviors have been integrated successfully, staff members' self-concept is enhanced, they are encouraged to trust that the system will support change efforts. These developments promote an openness to change both in the staff members and in the organization as a whole. In this stage, you work with the client to evaluate the overall success of the effort and develop a procedure for continued self-evaluation.

During each stage of the change process, the consultant works collaboratively with change sponsors, targets, advocates, and agents to identify and handle potential resistance to change.

Personal Resistance to Change

Resistance to change may come from a few individuals, in one or more work groups, or from the organizational culture as a whole. It is a normal phenomenon. Organizational responses to change are discussed in more detail below; personal responses to change are influenced by certain factors that determine the degree of resistance generated.

1. An individual's beliefs, attitudes, and values influence the way in which that individual perceives the self and the environment in relation to the self. They also affect the individual's ability to evaluate information from the environment objectively and act upon that information independently. The intensity with which beliefs, attitudes, and values are held is directly related to the individual's willingness to change in a given situation (Rokeach, 1960). If an

individual's strongly held beliefs, attitudes and values are incompatible with the organizational change, his or her resistance will be high. One of the benefits of change is that it forces us to evaluate old beliefs, attitudes, and values and adopt new ones where appropriate. If a change process gives participants the opportunity to explore these issues openly, their resistance is likely either to be diffused or to be recognized as a significant barrier that necessitates a reevaluation of the change effort.

2. The introduction of several changes within a short period can overwhelm staff members and increase their resistance to further changes. The number and pace of previous changes should be taken into account before any change effort is initiated.

3. A particular individual's resistance to change may be the result of changes in other life or work areas that have compromised his or her coping ability. Assess each person's readiness to undertake a change program, and build in support strategies if necessary.

4. As we noted earlier, recognition of a need for change is a prerequisite for willingness to change. To a large extent, you can prevent resistance to change by ensuring that all the staff members that will be affected by your intervention are aware of the need for change.

5. If previous changes have been unsuccessful or have created major crises because organizational support was not provided, staff members will be unwilling to go through the change process again, and their resistance will be high. Determine the type and amount of support needed, and make sure that it is available by the time the change process begins.

6. Individual fears, concerns, or problems with respect to a proposed change must be brought out into the open and managed in a way that reduces unnecessary stress. When this is not done, these feelings resurface as resistance at a later stage.

7. Change creates stress, and those individuals who are able to cope with work-related stress are also able to handle change relatively comfortably. When staff members have limited coping skills, or when a number of potential stressors are present, you must build coping strategies into the process of new skill development to enhance the commitment of the persons involved in the change.

8. Individuals with a strong internal locus of control (see chapter 2) are more likely to find opportunities in change and to believe in their ability to achieve goals when they can exercise some degree of control over those areas of the process that are important to them.

9. Creative thinkers are not tied to one way of looking at a problem; they are constantly finding new meanings and alternatives in the world around them. An innate desire to find new approaches increases receptiveness to change.

These nine factors determine the extent to which people will resist, withdraw, or commit themselves to a particular change project. Use Exercise 10.1 to determine how these factors are influencing the ways in which an individual or group with whom you are working responds to change.

Exercise 10.1 Personal Change Responses

Instructions. On the chart below, place a number on each arrow to indicate the degree to which each factor is influencing the responses of an individual or group to a current work change. Use a scale of 1 to 8, in which 1 = maximum resistance and 8 = maximum acceptance

Contributing Factor	Resistance/ Withdrawal 1	←→	Acceptance/ 8 Commitment
1	Threat to personal values or beliefs perceived	←→	No threat perceived or reclarified values congruent with change
2	Number or pace of changes induces sense of being overwhelmed	←→	Number and pace of changes are such that they can be absorbed
3	There are changes in other life/work areas occurring at the same time	←→	Other life changes are at a minimum
4	Need for change unclear	←→	Need for change clear
5	Low feeling of trust in support environment	←→	High trust in support environment

6	Feelings about change not addressed	⟷	Feelings about change accepted and addressed in some meaningful way
7	No or few personal coping skills	⟷	Coping skills high
8	External locus of control	⟷	Internal locus of control
9	Personal blocks to creative thinking	⟷	Pattern of creative thinking

Nursing and Change

As a nurse consultant, you have the opportunity to evaluate the impact that proposed changes will have on nurses and patient care. To make this evaluation, ask the following six critical questions.

1. To what extent will the proposed change facilitate or hinder the practice of professional nursing?
2. To what extent will the proposed change increase the patient's ability to achieve optimum health outcomes?
3. Are nurses aware of the need for change?
4. What are the sources of nurses' resistance to the change?
5. Do nurses have the skills necessary to make the change successfully?
6. On the basis of the answers to the previous five questions, what modifications or strategies should be incorporated into the change project?

The answers to these six questions, coupled with the information gained from Exercise 10.1, can be used to assess both the validity of a proposed change and the amount of resistance likely to be encountered during a change project. If resistance is coming from individuals or isolated groups in an organization, it is fairly easy to evaluate and manage; however, if it is an outgrowth of the organizational culture, an enormous amount of resources may be consumed in overcoming it.

ASSESSMENT OF ORGANIZATIONAL CULTURE

According to Conner (1985), "corporate culture is the basic pattern of shared beliefs, behaviors, and assumptions organization members acquire over time. . . . Assumptions are the unconscious rationale for continuing to apply certain beliefs or specific behaviors" (p. 2). Strong cultures are those that have a long tradition, stable membership, and a body of beliefs/behaviors/assumptions that are commonly held and formally and informally rewarded within the organization. Since strong cultures are not easily changed, any project must be evaluated in light of the relative strength of a given culture and the degree to which the change will disrupt that culture.

Your change proposals must include an analysis of the impact of the change on the existing culture. There are three questions that must be answered with respect to both the organizational culture and the nursing culture.

1. Is the organizational/nursing culture an appropriate one—that is, does it support the efforts the organization must make to be successful?
2. Is the organizational/nursing culture strong or weak?
3. Will the proposed changes disrupt the organizational/nursing culture?

When you have evaluated the appropriateness and strength of the culture and assessed the potential disruptive effects of suggested change strategies, one of four options is available to the client: (Conner, 1985).

1. If a major change will disrupt an inappropriate culture, you should alter the culture to support the change.
2. If a proposed minor change will reinforce an inappropriate culture or change it only minimally, you should consider aborting the change.
3. If a major change will modify an appropriate culture, you should modify the change itself to make it more consistent with the culture.
4. If a minor change is suggested that will have a minimal impact on the culture, you should not have high expectations for its potential beneficial effect, and you should reassess whether it is worth while to go ahead with the change.

If the client chooses to alter a strong culture, you must obtain clear answers to the following three questions.

1. Is the client aware of the resources, time, money, personnel, and active personal support needed for the project and willing to commit them to the project?
2. What modifications must be made in the culture to make it supportive of the change?
3. Do the change agents have the skills to modify the culture? If not, where will those skills be obtained?

Once these issues are resolved, you and your client are committed to a long-term effort. Strong cultures change slowly, if at all. In some cases major organizational restructuring and replacement of personnel have been necessary. The gains and losses of each change strategy must be carefully weighed.

Special Contribution of Nursing

Although nursing is clearly essential to the success of health-care organizations, too often these institutions employ consultants who have little or no understanding of the role of nursing and of the real needs of patients. Your unique perspective as a nurse consultant—the blend of organizational and nursing viewpoints—is the special vision that organizations need. The aim of the various examples in this chapter has been to show you how to integrate these two viewpoints in the context of a consulting endeavor. Armed with this knowledge, you will more easily be able to sort out the numerous organizational complexities you will encounter and restore organizations to a state of equilibrium. As you work within organizations, remember these six consulting guidelines.

1. Develop a framework for analyzing the complex layers of an organization's personality.
2. Identify the impact that a change will have on the culture of the organization and the impact that the culture will have on the change effort.
3. Integrate the various subsystems into the change.
4. Use the existing organizational resources whenever possible.
5. Remember that consulting is a collaborative process.
6. Develop your clients' skills so that they can continue to be successful when you leave.

Consulting offers nurses an additional avenue for growth and self-actualization. Chapters 9 and 10 have introduced you to the many exciting possibilities of this role. The books listed below contain additional information on consulting that will help you to develop new skills. As you attain greater proficiency as a nurse consultant, your increased ability to make a difference for nurses and clients will lead to a growing sense of achievement and self-esteem.

IV THE UNIQUE CONTRIBUTIONS OF NURSE ENTREPRENEURS

Many nurse entrepreneurs have been surprised by the negative and sometimes even hostile reactions of nursing colleagues to their entrepreneurial endeavors. They have been charged with a variety of crimes: treason, greed, withdrawal from the profession. In this final section, we lay these myths to rest by demonstrating the contributions that nurse entrepreneurs make to patients, nurses, and the profession.

11 ENHANCING NURSING THROUGH ENTREPRENEURSHIP

Nursing entrepreneurship affects not only the destiny of certain individual nurses, but also the way in which nursing as a whole is practiced. It expands the boundaries of nursing practice, and the results benefit patients, nurses, and the profession itself.

CONTRIBUTIONS TO PATIENTS

Nurse entrepreneurs intervene for patients as caregivers, as facilitators, and as advocates. An example of advocacy is provided by Dolores Alford, of the Institute of Gerontic Nursing, Inc.

> I was called to a nursing home to see a depressed, withdrawn, suicidal resident who went in and out of contact with reality. I talked with the woman, who felt useless. When I asked why, she burst into tears and said that she could no longer see. Her main joy in life was playing the piano, but now she could not read the notes. [Being] left alone in a darkened room made her do "funny things." I checked her eyes and found cataracts on each eye, even though her physical, done a month previously, showed no evidence of cataracts. I reported this to the physician, who was incensed that a nurse could use an ophthalmoscope. Even so, we arranged for surgery. Following surgery, she could see, play the piano, and was able to enjoy life again.

For Joan Dahlstedt, of Dahlstedt and Co, Inc, advocacy is a familiar component of nursing practice. She coordinates medical management for claims provided by insurance companies and uses her nursing judgement to make professional determinations about what is best for the patient.

> I have stopped unnecessary surgery and backed it up with a consult. I have been able to stop medications that were causing serious side effects and have been instrumental in getting patients off drugs that were incompatible with their other medications.

Nurses who own and manage businesses that provide health care bring a patient-centered approach to the industry that encourages advocacy on clients' behalf and client-centered solutions to health-care dilemmas. Sheila Felberbaum, of A Round The Clock Temporary Services, Inc, describes how she protected a patient from a potentially abusive situation.

> A patient receiving home care from us told her aide she was afraid of her caretaker. I contacted adult protective services, filed a complaint, had services increased to provide better supervision, and enforced protective supervision.

Marcia Harris, of Home Hospice Nursing, Inc, illustrates how nurses can make a difference for patients when they control health-care resources. Her corporation provides a broad spectrum of support to clients, including in-home skilled nursing care; volunteer emotional support and bereavement follow-up; consultative services in medicine, social work, pastoral care, and dietetics; and bedside care for up to 24 hours a day, if necessary. Her clients are adults and children with limited life expectancies.

> We were called to see a patient and family posing a problem for the HMO because of their daily irate phone calls and the perception that they were becoming antagonistic and difficult to work with. On my visit, I found a bedfast patient, dependent on continuous oxygen therapy, with draining lesions, moderate privacy needs, a deteriorating self-concept, loss of dignity, fear of dying, and fear of pain. I discovered a concerned and loving family, stressed by the patient's long illness and by their impending loss. Because of the hours the family members needed to work, the patient was left alone from 2 PM to 5 PM daily, a frightening experience for her. Currently, the patient was seen by a visiting nurse three times a week.
>
> I recommended: (1) drop the visiting nurse and supply an aide from 1:30 to 5:30 PM Monday through Friday (25% cost saving); (2) volunteer emotional support through a local hospice organization (no charge); (3) have her RN daughter ensure pain and symptom control with the physician; and (4) arrange future access, as needed, to nighttime patient assistance to allow the family rest/sleep prior to work days. The results of these changes were cost savings, decreased anger in the family, and the patient and family needs were met.

Another example of how nurses solve problems for their patients when they control the resources is provided by Barbara Bohny, of New Hope Respite and Home Care.

> A visiting health care agency consultated New Hope regarding the ways available to meet the needs of a client who did not qualify for their services. We were able to prevent institutionalizing the client by creating a unique plan of care implementing a respite care program.

Besides serving as patient advocates, problem solvers, and resource allocators, nurse entrepreneurs cut through the red tape of funding and regulations for their patients. Jamie Hills, of New Care Concepts, Inc, was able to perform this service for a client. New Care Concepts provides licensed nursing care for chronically ill or disabled children. One of their clients, a ventilator-dependent child, was living in a house with 18 steep steps. Family members and nursing staff had to carry the child, the wheelchair, and the ventilator (weighing a total of 225 pounds) up and down the stairs. For two years, the physician's request for a stair-trac device had been repeatedly turned down by the government provider. The family, unable to pay the $2,500 cost of the device, asked Hills for help.

> I consulted with my attorney, and both of us testified before the regulatory committee. We continued to write letters stating our case and pointing out the liability problem the state was creating for itself. We took a stand on the potential for injury our staff faced. It took four months, but the stair-trac was provided. To my knowledge, this is still a first; no one else has ever been approved.

Far from deserting clients, nurse entrepreneurs with greater autonomy and control over the resources clients need actually increase the options for these clients. The benefits of nurse entrepreneurship are not limited to patients but extend to nursing colleagues as well.

CONTRIBUTIONS TO NURSES AND NURSING

Patients and nurses alike gain from Dr. Dianne S. Moore's expertise. She is president of MOOREINFO, Inc, a company specializing in information on maternal-child health, women's health, obstetrics, midwifery, childbirth education, human sexuality, nursing, public health, research, and other areas on request. MOOREINFO's services include manuscript consultation, scientific research, grant writing, medical information provision, medical-legal research, continuing education, and patient care and education. Through this multifaceted business, she assists a wide variety of clients.

> I helped a doctoral student with her dissertation. She was really stuck and needed a fresh view on the topic and methodology. I also provided special classes, to prevent prematurity, to a woman on bedrest at home. She delivered on time and had a good labor and birth experience.

Donna Ipema, of Associates in Counseling, extends her expertise to colleagues in a comparable fashion.

> I worked with a nurse who was involved in power struggles with clients to uncover unresolved conflicts. As she learned to understand the reasons for her actions, she became a more effective nurse.

The contributions nurse entrepreneurs make to nursing include not only direct help but also information sharing and role modeling. Elizabeth Dayani uses all three of these avenues to assist other nurses. She formed American Nursing Resources Home Health Agency, Inc, in 1982. The corporation supplies supplemental staffing and home care by nurses, therapists, and nurse aides. In August 1987, she purchased Nurse-America, an agency that supplies nurses to areas throughout the country for temporary assignments. The wish to provide a role model was part of the stimulus for her decision to start a business.

> I wanted to prove that nurses could own and manage the business of nursing as well as or better than non-nurses. I speak locally and nationally, publish, and meet with and help nurses interested in going into business.

Ms. Dayani has also published an important and useful book, *The Nurse Entrepreneur* (Riccardi & Dayani, 1982). Through her example and personal efforts, she supports other nurses as they seek to expand their roles.

Another nurse entrepreneur who has provided valuable services to her colleagues is Dr. Vicki Lackman, of VL Associates. In addition to strengthening organizational and nursing effectiveness through her consultation and teaching, she works with nurses to help them manage personal stress. She has reached many nurses through her book, *Stress Management: A Manual For Nurses*. (Lachman, 1983)

Suzanne Hall Johnson, of Hall Johnson Communications, Inc, develops nurses' skills in a wide range of areas through her seminars, workshops, self-study modules, and publications. Through her efforts, nurses learn how to publish, how to start their own business, and how to improve their time management and marketing skills. In addition, she has enhanced the clinical practice of nursing as the editor of a critical care journal. In 1979, her book *High-Risk Parenting: Nursing Assessment and Strategies for the Family at Risk* (Johnson, 1979) received an AJN Book of the Year Award.

Two other nurses whose entrepreneurial roles have influenced nursing practice are Dr. Judith Pfister and Dr. Julia Kneedler, of Education Design, Inc. Through their business, Drs. Pfister and Kneedler provide consultation and educational programming and offerings for health-care providers, institutions, and industry. Many of their programs enhance nursing practice competencies.

> Members of Education Design have contributed in publishing, lecturing, and one-on-one with nurses in the clinical field and operating room. Dr. Judith Pfister has presented over 200 safety courses in clinical laser applications. Dr. Julia Kneedler has presented [courses on] perioperative nurse productivity, certification, and management.

So far, we have explored the contributions that nurse entrepreneurs who are in private practice, run an education-oriented business, or own a health-care provision business make to patients, nurses, and nursing practice. Nurses who are management consultants can make contributions of equal value. Joan Rizzi-Henderson, of JRH Associates, is a management consultant who works with hospital and nursing administrators to favorably alter the practice environment.

> I have helped nursing personnel bridge the gap between nursing practice and business concepts. For example, I was able to persuade a hospital administrator to increase the nursing budget by demonstrating the validity and reliability of the patient classification system.

This opportunity to improve the health-care environments in which nurses practice is present in many management consulting roles, as the following four examples indicate.

Jan Thornburg, of Professional Nurse Counselors, offers psychiatric mental health counseling in a manner that enhances both patient care and the nursing role.

> Acting as a consultant to a small private psychiatric hospital, I increase the knowledge of nursing administration and staff about treatment planning and the role of the nurse.

Karen Louise Christensen Hyland, of Professional Resources in Nursing, Inc, provides psychiatric mental health nursing to home-based patients; in addition, she is a nursing administration consultant and an educator. She integrates these roles to upgrade practice environments—for example, by helping a facility prepare and pass a JCAH accreditation process. Improving the environment in health-care organizations increases the opportunities for quality nursing practice and quality patient care.

Dominick S. Cullen, of CAI Management Systems, combines his 28 years of experience in nursing and nursing management with an in-depth knowledge of computers in his consulting business. Among the contributions he has made to nursing is "achieving a reduction in staffing costs while maintaining a high level of care using a computer staffing system."

Some nurse entrepreneurs have an impact on a total health-care delivery process. Michael Johnson, of Consulting Opinion, Inc, feels that his services both upgrade the system and improve access to health care.

> My services as a program developer, lecturer, and trainer have improved the quality and access of home care and aging services in the community. I have helped organizations by designing the operational guidelines and by assisting them to comply with regulations when deficiencies are present.

Nurse entrepreneurs are creating practice opportunities for all nurses. The chance to make a difference professionally can be a powerful stimulus for other nurses to try their hands at entrepreneurship.

CONCLUSION: THE FUTURE OF NURSE ENTREPRENEURS

Nurse entrepreneurs are here to stay. Not every nurse will choose this role, but all nurses and patients will benefit from the endeavors of those who do. As nurse entrepreneurs enable and empower themselves, they simultaneously enable and empower nurses and patients. As they exercise more control over their practice and the health-care resources needed by patients, they increase the choices available to patients, and they make it possible for nurses in traditional practice environments to become more intrapreneurial. Nurse entrepreneurs are not leaving nursing; rather, they are expanding its boundaries and creating new options for nurses and clients alike.

Entrepreneurship gives nurses a choice, a new avenue for practice. Our goals in writing this book have been (1) to provide potential entrepreneurs with the information, skills, and resources they need to make the change, and (2) to increase all nurses' understanding of the entrepreneurial role itself. Whichever nursing career path you choose, an entrepreneurial orientation opens doors and creates opportunities for autonomy, independence, and professional fulfillment. Therefore, we close this book with an entrepreneurial wish: may you discover limitless opportunities to expand your nursing role, and may you find the professional networks to support your endeavors.

REFERENCES

Aldrich, N. W. (1986, June). p. 65 Young founders. *Inc.*

Aslett, D. (1986, August 20). How much work do men do? In Cruver, D., Husbands and housework: It's still an uneven load. *USA Today*, p. 5 D.

Ballas, G. C., & Hollas, D. (1980). *The making of an entrepreneur: Keys to your success*. Englewood Cliffs, NJ: Prentice-Hall.

Baty, G. B. (1974). *Entrepreneurship: Playing to win*. Reston, VA: Reston.

Bell, C., & Nadler, L. (1985). *Clients and consultants*. Houston: Gulf.

Birch, D. L. (1987, September). The rise and fall of everybody. *INC.*, pp. 18, 19, 21.

Blake, R., & Mouton, J. (1983). *Consultation*. (2nd ed.). Reading, MA: Addison-Wesley.

Block, P. (1981). *Flawless consulting: A guide to getting your expertise used*. San Diego: University Associates.

Bloom, P. N. (1984, September–October). Marketing for professional services. *Harvard Business Review*, (5), 102.

Bolles, R. N. (1986). *The 1986 what color is your parachute?* Berkeley, CA: Ten Speed Press.

Broom, H. N., Longenecker, J. & Moore, C. W. (1983). *Small-business management* (6th ed.). Cincinnati: South-Western.

Church, O. D. (1984). *Small business management and entrepreneurship*. Chicago: Science Research Associates.

Connelly, M. (1986, May 19). p 27. Strength in Numbers. *Wall Street Journal* p. 27.

Conner, D. R. (1985). *The culture audit workbook: Corporate culture and its impact on organizational change*. Atlanta: OD Resources, Inc.

Connor, R. A., Jr., & Davidson, J. P. (1985). *Marketing your consulting and professional services*. New York: John Wiley & Sons.

Cook, J. (1986). *The start-up entrepreneur*. New York: Truman Talley.

Cruver, D. (1986, August 20), Husbands and housework: It's still an uneven load. *USA Today*, p. 5D.

Deal, T. E., & Kennedy, A. A. (1982). *Corporate cultures: The rites and rituals of corporate life*. Reading, MA: Addison-Wesley.

Doleysh, N. (1986). The consultant's role in enhancing practice skills. *Nursing Administration Quarterly, 10* (4), p. 82–83.

Drucker, P. E. (1967). *The effective executive*. New York: Harper and Row.

Drucker P. E. (1984, January–February). Our entrepreneurial economy. *Harvard Business Review, 1* (6), 58.

Drucker, P. E. (1985). *Innovation and entrepreneurship: Practice and principles*. New York: Harper and Row.

Edmunds, S. W. (1982). *Performance measures for growing businesses*. New York: Van Nostrand Reinhold.

Eisenhauer, L. A. (1986, October). Health care brokering—a career option for changing times. *Nursing & Health Care, 7* (8), 417.

Fieve, R. (1987, February). The manic-depressive entrepreneur. *Success!*, p. 56.

Frame, R. M., Hess, R. K., & Nielsen, W. R. (1982). *The OD source book: A practitioner's guide*. San Diego: University Associates.

Fritz, R. (1987). *Nobody gets rich working for somebody else: An entrepreneur's guide*. New York: Dodd, Mead and Company.

Gilder, G. (1984). *The spirit of enterprise*. New York: Simon and Schuster.

Goldstein, H. A. (1985). *One hundred and twenty-two minutes a month to greater profits*. Los Angeles: Granville.

Gray, D. A. (1985). *Start and run a profitable consulting business*. Seattle: Self-Counsel Press.

Hartman, C. (1986, June). Main Street, Inc. *INC.*, p. 54.

Hartley, R. F. (1986). *Marketing mistakes* (3rd ed.). New York: John Wiley & Sons.

Holland, P. (1984). *The entrepreneur's guide*. New York: Penguin.

Hymowitz, C. & Schellhardt, T. (1986, March 24). The glass ceiling. *Wall Street Journal*, p. 1.

Johnson, S. H. (1979). *High risk parenting: Nursing assessment and strategies for the family at risk*. New York: J. B. Lippincott.

Kelley, R. E. (1981). *Consulting: The complete guide to a profitable career*. New York: Scribner.

Kirzner, I. M. (1979). *Perception, opportunity, and profit*. Chicago: University of Chicago Press.

Kotler, P. (1986). *Principles of marketing* (3rd ed.). Englewood Cliffs, NJ: Prentice-Hall.

Lachman, V. C. (1983). *Stress management: A manual for nurses*. San Diego: Grune and Stratton.

Lange, F. C. (1987). *The nurse as an individual, group, or community consultant*. Norwalk, CT: Appleton-Century-Crofts.

Levinson, J. C. (1984). *Guerilla marketing*. Boston: Houghton Mifflin.

Lippit, G., & Lippit, R. (1978). *The consulting process in action*. San Diego: University Associates.

Mancuso, J. R. (1984). *How to start, finance, and manage your own small business* (rev. ed.). Englewood Cliffs, NJ: Prentice-Hall.

Mancuso, J. R. (1987, April). Testing your hunches. *Success!*, p.6.

McClelland, D. C. (1967). p. 211 *The achieving society: Characteristics of entrepreneurship*. Princeton, NJ: D. Van Nostrand Company.

Merrill, R. E., & Sedwick, H. D. (1987). *The new venture handbook*. New York: AMACOM.

Milhaven, A. (1984). p. 48 Professional for-profit corporations balance the market for nursing services. *Nursing Management, 15* (3).

Naisbitt, J. (1984). p. 17,261 *Megatrends*. New York: Warner Communications.

The New Business Guide (1986). Prepared by the Milwaukee Department of City Development, Division of Economic Development. Milwaukee, WI.

Nobel, B. P. (1986, July). A sense of self. *Venture*, p. 36.

Pareek, U. (1982). Internal and external control. In *The 1982 annual for facilitators, trainers, and consultants*. San Diego: University Associates.

Rao, T. V. (1985). The entrepreneurial orientation inventory: measuring the locus of control. In Goodstein, L. D., & Pfeiffer, J. W. (Eds.), *The 1985 annual: Developing human resources* (pp. 129–137). San Diego: University Associates, 1985.

Riccardi, B. R. & Dayani, E. C. (1982). *The nurse entrepreneur*. Reston, VA: Reston.

Rodale, J. I. (1978). *The synonym finder*. New York: Warner Books.

Rokeach, M. (1960). *The open and closed mind*. New York: Basic Books.

Schein, E. (1969). *Process consultation: Its role in organizational development*. Reading, MA: Addison-Wesley.

Shornes, L. (1986, June 8). Wharton reaches for the stars. *The New York Times Magazine: Pt. 2. p. 84, The Business World*.

Silvester, J. L. (1984). *How to start, finance and operate your own business*. Secaucus, NJ: Lyle Stuart.

Solis, D. (1986, March 24). p. 24D Family practices. *Wall Street Journal*.

Welsh, J. A., & White, J. F. (1983). *The entrepreneur's master planning guide: How to launch a successful business*. Englewood Cliffs, NJ: Prentice-Hall.

White, R. M. (1977). *The entrepreneur's manual*. Radnor, PA: Chilton.

Women Entrepreneurs: The new business owners. (1986, July). *Venture*, p. 35.

Wojahn, E. (1986, July). p. 46 Why aren't there more women in this magazine? *Inc.*

1986: Year of the woman entrepreneur. (1986, January). p. 35 *Working Woman*.

Appendix A NURSE ENTREPRENEURS WHO CONTRIBUTED TO THIS BOOK

We extend our warmest thanks to the nurse entrepreneurs listed below, who contributed their experiences and insights to this book by answering our questionnaire and responding to our telephone questions. Their participation in the project transformed it into a celebration of a new spirit of independence in nurses.

American Nursing Associates
Susan L. Reuler
Executive Director
S. 250 Leetsdale Drive, #125
Denver, CO 80222
(303) 393-0600

AMERICAN NURSING RESOURCES HOME HEALTH AGENCY, INC.
Elizabeth Dayani, RNC, MSN,
Corporate Administrator
11050 Roe Boulevard, Suite 200
Overland Park, KS 66211
(913) 491-0010; (800) 333-3369

AMK ASSOCIATES
Alice-Marie Kotkowski, RN
President
23 East Washington Street
Chicago, IL 60602
(312) 664-7630

Andicore, Inc.
Norma L. Lewis, PhD, RN
PO Box 54
Liberty, MO 64068
(816) 792-0154

A Round The Clock Temporary Services, Inc.
Sheila B. Felberbaum
344 Deer Park Avenue
PO Box 548
Babylon, NY 11702
(516) 669-4141

Associates in Counseling
Donna K. Ipema
6601 W. College Drive
Palos Heights, IL 60463
(312) 597-3000, ext. 335

Eileen K. Austin, Inc.
PO Box 168
Crystal Beach, FL 34256
(813) 786-5557

BJC & Associates
Barbara J. Chadwick
14527 Redbud Trail N.
Buchanan, MI 41907
(616) 695-2166

Nikki Brierton, MS, RN
40 W. 77th Street
New York, NY 10024
(212) 798-2657

CAI Management Systems
Dominick J. Cullen, RN
PO Box 864
Calhoun, GA 30701
(404) 625-2378

Consulting Opinion, Inc.
Michael Johnson
President
375 NE 163rd
Seattle, WA 98155

CPR Associates
Laura Gasparis, MA, RN, CEN, CCRN
130 Delafield Avenue
Staten Island, NY 10301
(718) 727-5414

Dahlstedt & Company, Inc.
Joan Dahlstedt
301 W. Osborn
Suite 105
Phoenix, AZ 85013
(602) 263-8951

Delaware Nursing Centers, Inc.
Salle McDaniel, BSN, RN
24 Holly Way
Riverwoods
Wilmington, DE 19809
(302) 762-8644

Diabetic Shoppe
Connie Roethal
5530 N. Port Washington Road
Milwaukee, WI 53217
(414) 963-1939

DOWNTOWN WOMEN'S CENTER
Cynthia Casoff, CNM
Director
412 Avenue of the Americas (3rd floor)
New York, NY 10011
(212) 529-7722

Education Design, Inc.
Judith L. Pfister, President
5925 E. Evans Avenue
Suite 202C
Denver, CO 80222
(303) 692-9758

FAMILY HEALTH CARE, INC.
Carolyn Edison
PO Box 205
Liberty, MI 64068
(815) 781-3202

Delores M. Giltner
925 Main Street A
Broomfield, CO 80020
(303) 469-5754

Giltner Enterprises
Delores M. Giltner
229 Retail Center, Suite 119
Broomfield, CO 80020
(303) 469-5325

Hall Johnson Communications, Inc.
Suzanne Hall Johnson, MSN, RN
Director
9737 W. Ohio Avenue
Lakewood, CO 80226

Haller's Nursing Care, Inc.
Carol L. Haller
3601 Adobe Street
Evansville, IN 47712
(812) 428-0678

Health Care Consultants of Wisconsin
Judy Dean
N64 W26303 Hillview Drive
Sussex, WI 53089
(414) 246-8611

Health Care Professionals, Ltd.
Adeline A. Laforet
17000 W. 8 Mile, Suite 350
Southfield, MI 48075
(313) 423-6500

Health Savers, Inc.
Edna A. Lauterbach
419 Route 9W North
Newburgh, NY 12550
(914) 561-9300

Home Hospice Nursing, Inc.
Marcia Harris, MS, RN
880 S. Catherine
LaGrange, IL 60525
(312) 482-4550

Humanistic Programming & Planning
GENEIE Everett Fellows, RN
419 Sycamore, NE
Albuquerque, NM 87106
(505) 843-6033

Independent Nursing Services
Susan R. Donaldson
Box 1192
Oil City, PA 16301
(412) 647-4497

INSTITUTE OF GERONTIC NURSING INC,
Dolores M. Alford
8215 Westchester Drive, Suite 131
Dallas, TX 75225
(214) 691-0717

Lorraine Jacobson of Wingspan
13228 Marine Drive
Marysville, WA 98270
(206) 643-7074

JRH Associates
Joan Rizzi-Henderson
15 Sunset Drive
Weston, CT 06883
(203) 226-8103

Barbara Klein, RN, CRC, CIRS
Rehabilitation Coordinator
PO Box 2264
Capistrano Beach, CA 92624
(714) 493-2534

Laconia Women's Health Care
Nancy E. Dirubbo
366 Union Avenue
Laconia, NH 03246
(603) 528-4304

Management & Career Resources
Carole Meola
St. Paul Building, Suite 600
125 St. Paul's Boulevard
Norfolk, VA 23510-2710
(804) 627-2682, ext. 65

MOOREINFO INC.
Dianne S. Moore, PhD, CNM
54 Butterwood Lane, NW
Irvington-On-Hudson, NY 10533
(914) 591-6748

MOSS BAY PREVENTIVE MEDICINE
Barb Dalpez
607 Market
Kirkland, WA 98033
(206) 822-9559

Nelson Institute
Joan L. Nelson
1010 North Orchard
Boise, ID 83706
(308) 377-8204

NEW CARE CONCEPTS, INC.
Jamie Hills
2208 NW Market, #302
Seattle, WA 98107
(206) 789-9054

New Hope Respite & Home Care
Barbara J. Bohny, RN, DNS
8 Summit Avenue
Haledon, NJ 07508
(201) 956-1264

NORTHWEST NEIGHBORHOOD NURSES, INC.
Andrea Karlin
Executive Director
1819 NW Everett
Portland, OR 97209
(503) 224-3107 (O); (503) 224-0289 (clinic)

Nurse Care, Ltd.
Ann Butts, RN
302 Triune Mill Road
Thomaston, GA 30286
(404) 647-9523

Nurse Counseling Group
Lenore U. Boles, MS, RN, CS
Linda L. Hackett, MA, RN CS
114 East Avenue
Norwalk, CT 06851
(202) 838-1678

NURSE EDU-CARE RESOURCE NETWORK (NEC/RN)
Penny Hamlin, BA, RN
Jane Aral, BA, MEd, RN
430 S. Union Avenue
Alliance, OH 44601
(216) 821-3635

NURSE PRACTITIONER ASSOCIATES
R. Mimi Clarke Secor, MEd, RNC, FNP
2464 Massachusetts Avenue
Cambridge, MA 02140
(617) 354-6028

Nurses in Transition
Dianne Duchesne
Executive Director
85 Wood Land
Fairfax, CA 94930
(414) 453-2360

NURSING ASSOCIATES
Dolores M. Alford, MSN, RN, FANN
Janet A. Moll, MS, RN, GNP
8215 Westchester Drive
Suite 131
Dallas, TX 75225
(214) 691-0717

NU-VISION, INC.
Carolyn H. Brose, EdD, RN
Box 551
Liberty, MO 64068
(816) 792-0154

Margaret Y. O'Brien, Inc.
HEALTH CARE CONSULTANTS
17490 Timberleigh Way
Woodbine, MD 21797
(301) 854-6041

Donna Oram
309 E 68 Terrace
Kansas City, MO 64113
(816) 561-0080

Professional Nurse Counselors
Jan Thornburg, MS, RNCS
2201 San Pedro, NE
Building #2, Suite 222
Albuquerque, NM 87110
(505) 266-6060

Professional Nursing Associates
Susan L. Reuler
President
S. 250 Leetsdale Drive, #125
Denver, CO 80222
(303) 393-0600

Professional Resources in Nursing, Inc.
Karen Louise Christensen Hyland
12715 Mohawk CR
Leawood, KS 66209
(913) 491-3147

Louise Ransed
801 Springdale Avenue
Annapolis, MD 21403
(301) 263-0375

Ruth's Maternity/GYN Clinic
Ruth V. Halvorson, ARNP, CNM
321 E. Division
Mount Vernon, WA 98273
(206) 336-6683

SCE
Self Care Education
Janice Crist, MS, RN
PO Box 7633
Olympia, WA 98507-7633
(206) 943-7624

Stone & Associates
Mary Ellen Stone, BSN, RN
139 Lake Drive
Stanhope, NJ 07874
(201) 347-5087

Candice Telis, EdD, RN, CS
2 Main Street
Hennington, NJ 08822
(201) 782-1727

VL ASSOCIATES
Vicki D. Lachman, PhD, RN
150 N. Second Street
Philadelphia, PA 19106
(215) 627-8425

J.C. WARDEN & ASSOCIATES
Joan C. Warden, BSN, RN
President
Reed Hartman Corporate Center
10999 Reed Hartman Highway
Cincinnati, OH 45242
(513) 791-3679

THE WARMING TOUCH
Joell E. Archibald, BSN, MBA, RNC
4315 57th Street Court E.
Tacoma, WA 98443
(206) 922-9086

Karen Bonnell Wern, MS, ARNP
10604 NE 38th Place
Suite 114
Kirkland, WA 98033
(206) 454-4510

WHEELER & ASSOCIATES
Sheila Quilter Wheeler, MA, RN
President
508 San Anselmo Boulevard, #18
San Anselmo, CA 94960
(415) 453-8382

Patricia C. Wilson, RN
1110 Charmuth Road
Lutherville, MD 21093
(301) 821-7526

Appendix B BUSINESS PLAN: WORKING COPY

This is your opportunity to use the content and exercises in chapters 3 through 8 to prepare a working copy of a business plan. Be specific and succinct. To encourage brevity, we have purposely specified the number of pages to be used to complete certain sections. Potential investors prefer facts without adornment. Remembers, this is a rough draft, not the finished project.

If you wish, you may reproduce part or all of this appendix for your own use.

Instructions. Follow these 17 steps to complete the working copy of your business plan.

1. Complete the cover page (p. B5)
2. Complete market research and analysis (pp. B15–B17)
3. Complete the marketing plan (pp. B18–B20)
4. Complete your financial plan (pp. B30, B31)
5. Describe your company (pp. B11, B12)
6. Describe the industry (pp. B13, B14)
7. Describe the management team (pp. B21, B22)
8. Describe the support team (p. B23)
9. Complete the operations plan (pp. B24, B25)
10. Describe your research and development plan (p. B26)
11. Describe your overall schedule (pp. B27, B28)
12. List critical risks and problems (p. B29)
13. Discuss your proposed financing (p. B32)
14. Describe the legal structure of the company (p. B33)
15. Complete the executive summary (pp. B6–B8)
16. Compile the appendices and supporting documents (pp. B33+)
17. Complete the table of contents (pp. B9, B10)

Now review and refine your plan and prepare a high-quality document to present to your expert adviser or your banker. They will tell you if additions to the plan are necessary. If you do not require expert advice or financial services, use this plan as a guide for your start-up period. Work on developing an effective personal presentation of the plan. Your ability to attract clients and investors depends on your ability to sell the business concept contained in this plan.

COVER PAGE

Company name:

Address:

Telephone:

Date:

Name(s) of principal(s):

EXECUTIVE SUMMARY

In the next three pages or less, briefly describe your company's product/ service, the unique factors that distinguish you from the competition, your marketability, and your business objectives. Discuss the management of the business; summarize your financial projections; and identify the amount, sources, and purposes of the money required for the business.

(executive summary continued)

(executive summary continued)

TABLE OF CONTENTS

List and describe the major sections of the plan. Include a brief description of the contents of each section, and indicate the page numbers.

(table of contents continued)

DESCRIPTION OF COMPANY

In two pages or less, describe your business, the product/service you provide, your potential clients, what specific needs you are meeting, the competitive advantage you have, and your potential markets for the business in the future. Discuss how you will reach customers and how they will reach you. Describe the image your company will have.

(description of company continued)

DESCRIPTION OF INDUSTRY

In two pages or less, briefly describe the dominant trends in the industry that are shaping the market for your business now and in the future. List your sources of information.

(description of industry continued)

MARKET RESEARCH AND ANALYSIS

This is the first step in business planning and the most critical one: the demonstration that there is a market for your products/services. In the next three pages, indicate your data sources, your specific market segments, the relevant market trends, and the size of your markets. Identify your competitors, their current strength, their likely response to your entering the market, and the features that distinguish your products/services from theirs. Identify your market geographically: Where will you do business? What is the size of the market? What share of the market will you have? What will you charge? What are your market share projections for the next one, five, and ten years? What are your revenue projections? Review the discussion of market testing in chapter 3 to help you complete this section.

(market research and analysis continued)

(market research and analysis continued)

MARKETING PLAN

In three pages, list your marketing goals and discuss the strategies you will use to reach each of your target markets. Identify the persons accountable for marketing; indicate the cost of each strategy; and describe how you will monitor emerging markets and evaluate how well current marketing strategies are working. Refer to chapter 6 for help if necessary.

(marketing plan continued)

(marketing plan continued)

MANAGEMENT TEAM

In this and the following page, outline the management team. Draw an organizational chart, and include a job description for each management position. Discuss the competencies, experience, and credentials that each key management person brings to the team. (Include in the appendix.) Discuss compensation, ownership privileges, profit sharing, and other issues as they apply to key management personnel. If you have a board of directors, describe the expertise that each member brings to the management team and the role that the board plays in the corporation.

(management team continued)

SUPPORT TEAM

Describe the expert services (e.g., accounting, financial, legal, and technical) that you will utilize to develop and maintain a successful business.

OPERATIONS PLAN

Describe how you will organize the work process. Include information about personnel, location, equipment, and other essential operational elements. Discuss the work to be done, who will do the work, and the time and money required to accomplish the work. Review chapter 5 for assistance with this part of the business plan.

(operations plan continued)

RESEARCH AND DEVELOPMENT PLAN

Discuss your plans for research and development to secure the future of your business. How much time, energy, and money will be devoted to this effort?

OVERALL SCHEDULE

Identify the timetable for critical activities both before and after the start-up period. These activities might include locating an office space, hiring personnel, or contacting the first client.

Critical Activity	Month

(overall schedule continued)

Critical Activity	Month

CRITICAL RISKS AND PROBLEMS

Discuss the major risks and problems you face, and explain your strategies for dealing with them.

FINANCIAL PLAN

1. On the next page, discuss your financial plan, using information derived from the exercises in chapter 7.
2. Add a section on "supporting financial documentation", which should include the following:
   A. a company budget, with at least a one-year projection;
   B. start-up balance sheet and income projection statement (if you have an existing business, include copies of each of these documents for the semiannual periods of the first year and for annual periods in succeeding years);
   C. a cash-flow projection for at least one year (you may be requested to submit a three-year projection if you are seeking additional financing for the business;
   D. a budget deviation analysis for each month you are in business; and
   E. a break-even analysis.

(financial plan and supporting documentation continued)

PROPOSED FINANCING

Outline your plan for obtaining the necessary financing for the business. How much money will you require, and for what purposes? What will you invest? Where will you obtain additional funds? Include a personal financial statement if you intend to find outside capital.

LEGAL STRUCTURE

Describe the legal structure of your business.

Appendix C SAMPLE PROJECT PROPOSAL FOR A HOSPITAL

Analysis/Discussion of Client Need. As per our discussion of 8/26/86, the purpose of this project is to establish a solid foundation for orthopaedic nursing (including skills, theory, standards of care, policies, and procedures) for selected nursing staff at __________ Hospital. The major goals that this project will accomplish are (1) increased nursing staff proficiency in caring for the level of orthopaedic patients currently served and (2) development of a foundation of skill and theory that will serve as the basis of nursing care in the provision of care to patients with complex orthopaedic needs.

Preliminary Program Design. The achievement of the goals stated above will be accomplished most effectively in the manner described below.

Time	Activity
3.5 hours	1. Exploratory/explanatory meetings with nursing and medical staff to explain project, answer questions, receive suggestions, establish working relationship.
10.0 hours	2.a. Assessment of current status. Review of documents directing and recording care: orthopedic specialty sheets (CMS and traction check, for example), nursing care plans, nursing diagnosis format, nursing care standards, patient teaching materials.
4.5 hours	2.b. Assessment of available in-house resources: equipment, library, audiovisuals, personnel.
6.5 hours	2.c. Assessment of nursing staff. This phase involves development and administration of a tool for assessing nurses' perceptions of their own knowledge and needs. An objective determination of their orthopaedic knowledge will also be obtained via the development and administration of a pretest.
4.5 hours	3. Analyze results of assessment to identify learning needs. Determine discrepancies

between perceptual and actual knowledge base. Refer those problems that are amenable to managerial strategies to management. Develop educational strategies to resolve knowledge deficits

14.0 hours	4. Prepare instructional format. Develop objectives. Determine learning experiences needed. Develop content plans. Investigate availability of appropriate audiovisuals; order books; designate appropriate personnel as clinical preceptors and classroom instructors. Meet with all teaching personnel to ensure internal consistency in approach and content provided to staff in classroom and clinical learning experiences. Obtain input and develop schedule for learning activities. Ensure that all arrangements—for videotaping equipment, slide presentation, movie or slide projectors, room assignments, refreshments, etc.,—have been accomplished.
72.0 hours	5. Clinical/role modeling. Arrange time and dates for six four-hour sessions on each shift for direct contact with individual staff nurses. These sessions will provide opportunities for one-to-one interaction, which is beneficial in enhancing and developing specialty nursing clinical decision-making/patient care skills.
240.0 hours	6. Classroom instruction. A total of 80 hours is allotted to direct classroom contact. Remaining time is spent on development of handouts, outlines, quizzes, review of videotapes for accuracy and clarity, and application for ANA-recognized continuing education units (if desired), among other activities.

As per our discussion, specific content to be included in classroom presentation includes

- physical and psychologic assessment of the orthopaedic patients,
- emergency and intensive care of the patient with a spinal cord injury,
- integrating care of orthopedic injuries into the total care plan for a critically ill or traumatized patient,
- motorcycle trauma, and
- intraoperative care of the orthopedic patient,

16.5 hours

7. Final test. Test is prepared, administered, and corrected; results are collated; feedback is provided to group; and recommendations are generated.

8.0 hours

8. Communication with staff nurses and doctors. In addition to the introductory/explanatory time in activity 1, eight hours of verbal and written communication time are built into the project. This provides the time necessary for investigating problems, answering questions, and complying with requests for assistance with special needs.

48.0 hours

9. Committee work and team building. This time is needed to build an orthopaedic team that will serve as the nucleus for development of solutions to future and ongoing nurse practice needs. The team will be prepared to deal with standards of nursing care with patients of increased complexity, nursing forms, teaching tools, policies, and procedures. In addition to the contribution made to departmental management, these activities contribute to staff's sense of achievement and recognition, thereby improving motivation and productivity. This approach to

	orthopaedic content also makes it impossible for the departure of one staff member to take away all the institution's orthopedic expertise. Projects of other sorts (quality assurance, for example) can be assigned to the team as a working group, or the team can be used as a model to spread this approach to other in-house projects. The early sessions are aimed at encouraging group/team development, offering technical assistance, providing expert input, and supporting group and change process.
32.0 hours	10. Review of committee-developed output. Evaluation, recommendations, input, reinforcement, encouragement, and support are provided.
10.0 hours	11. Interim progress reports and strategy meetings with nursing adminstration. These communication efforts, amounting to ten hours spread throughout the project, will direct the course of the project.
10.5 hours	12. Termination of consulting relationship. This final phase involves reviewing progress, preparing a final report, and meeting to present the final report and recommendations. If desired, preparation and presentation of CEU certificates can be included here. This phase could logically include assistance with development and implementation of strategies to recoup return on investment.
480.0 hours total @ $50.00/hour = $24,000.00, plus expenses. Project to be accomplished over a four-month period.	

Proposer's Qualifications Relevant to Project Requirements. *Educational qualifications*—double major in a master's program; nursing education and clinical specialty.

Experiential qualifications—staff nurse in orthopaedics, assistant director of nursing in charge of orthopaedics, assistant professor of nursing in charge of teaching classroom and clinical senior medical-surgical component in orthopaedics, orthopaedic clinical nurse specialist, currently trauma nurse specialist (large orthopaedic injury population) with fire department rescue squad, national and international lecturer on orthopaedics.

Orthopaedic publications—"Holistic rehabilitation of the patient with low back pain." Wisconsin Orthopaedic Nurses Association Educational Newsletter, Spring 1983.

Neuromuscular Section Editor and Contributor to *Core Curriculum for Orthopaedic Nursing*. Pitman, NJ: Anthony J. Jannetti, 1986.

Doleysh, N. C. (in press). Musculoskeletal problems: Joint disorders. In *NurseReview*, Springhouse, PA: Springhouse.

Award in Orthopaedics—1979–1980 Senior Students' Award for Outstanding Clinical and Classroom Teacher at Marquette University.

1986 National Orthopaedic Nurses Association Certificate of Appreciation for Outstanding Service.

Appendix D SAMPLE LETTER OF INTENT

WORKSTYLES

2205 East Menlo Boulevard
Shorewood, WI 53211
Phone: (414) 332-1202

July 18, 1985

XXXXXX XXXXXX
Vice President, Nursing
XXXXXXX XXXXX Hospital
XXXXXXXXXXXXXXX
XXXXXXXXXXXXXX

Dear XXXXXXXX,

This letter confirms our agreement for my consulting services discussed during our June 12 meeting.

Project. I will hold six team building sessions with your management team on the dates listed below.

Purpose. The purpose of these sessions is to assist team members to identify a common focus; develop procedures for effective problem solving; identify guidelines for conflict management and feedback; negotiate leadership roles within the group; and plan for ongoing team development.

Objectives. During these sessions, members will:

1. identify the purpose, values, and goals of the nursing management team,
2. describe the specific strengths that each person brings to the work of the team,
3. examine how leadership roles are filled within the group,
4. develop specific guidelines for conflict management and negative feedback among team members,
5. establish problem-solving strategies the team will use in decision making.

6. clarify power-sharing strategies that allow each member to fulfill role expectations,

7. negotiate the mutual expectations that the team manager and members have of each other,

8. integrate these strategies into the team interactions between sessions, and

9. develop a plan to evaluate team progress at specific intervals in order to continue the growth process.

Schedule

DATE	SESSION	CONTENT	TIME: 1 PM– 4 PM
	1	Team purpose and goals, strengths and roles of members	3 hours
	2	Negotiating leadership roles	3 hours
	3	Developing guidelines for conflict management and providing feedback	3 hours
	4	Group problem-solving strategies: decision making, decision evaluation and decision support	3 hours
	5	Power management: exploring ways in which power can be used to benefit the group	3 hours
	6	Team development: evaluating process, resetting goals	3 hours

There will be a total of 18 contact hours with the management team. After the last session, I will prepare a written report that includes an analysis of the status of team development and suggested strategies for continued self-assessment and development. I will review the report with you during a one-hour meeting to be scheduled within three weeks of the final team building session.

Participants at the sessions will include yourself, your two assistants, and the eight area managers.

Fee. My fee for the project is $1,500. $750 will be paid within two weeks of the third session, and the remainder will be paid within two weeks of our final meeting.

This contract may be terminated by written notice provided two weeks in advance of any scheduled session. In case of termination before project completion, I will bill you for hours of contact at the rate of $85.00 per hour.

Your signature at the bottom of this letter will constitute an agreement for this project as described. Please sign and return one copy to me, and retain one for your records.

I look forward to working with your management team.

Sincerely,

Gerry Vogel, MSN, RN
Director, WORKSTYLES

This letter constitutes our agreement for the team building project described at the fee indicated.

Date: ____________________ ____

XXXXXX XXXXX
Vice president, nursing

Appendix E SAMPLE FORMAL CONTRACT FOR ON-SITE CONSULTING/ CONTINUING EDUCATION

Agreement Between Hospital and Advanced Health Care Concepts. The following description of consulting/continuing education services and fees herein represents the sum total of agreement between the two parties.

Time	Activity
3.5 hours	1. Exploratory/explanatory meetings with nursing and medical staff to explain project, answer questions, receive suggestions, establish working relationship.
10.0 hours	2.a. Assessment of current status. Review of documents directing and recording care: orthopedic specialty sheets (CMS and traction check, for example), nursing care plans, nursing diagnosis format, nursing care standards, patient teaching materials.
4.5 hours	2.b. Assessment of available in-house resources: equipment, library, audiovisuals, personnel.
6.5 hours	2.c. Assessment of nursing staff. This phase involves development and administration of a tool for assessing nurses' perceptions of their own knowledge and needs. An objective determination of their orthopedic knowledge will be obtained via the development and administration of a pretest.
4.5 hours	3. Analyze results of assessment to identify learning needs. Determine discrepancies between perceptual and actual knowledge base. Refer those problems that are amenable to managerial strategies to management. Develop educational strategies to resolve knowledge deficits.
14.0 hours	4. Prepare instructional format. Develop objectives. Determine learning experiences needed. Develop content

plans. Investigate availability of appropriate audiovisuals; order books; designate appropriate personnel as clinical preceptors and classroom instructors. Meet with all teaching personnel to ensure internal consistency in approach and content provided to staff in classroom and clinical learning experiences. Obtain input and develop schedule for all learning activities. Ensure that all arrangements—for videotaping equipment, slide preparation, movie or slide projectors, room assignments, refreshments, etc.—have been accomplished.

72.0 hours

5. Clinical/role modeling. Arrange times and dates for six four-hour sessions on each shift for direct contact with individual staff nurses. These sessions will provide opportunities for one-to-one interaction, which is beneficial in enhancing and developing specialty nursing clinical decision-making/patient care skills.

240.0 hours

6. Classroom instruction. A total of 80 hours is allotted to direct classroom contact. Remaining time is spent on development of handouts, outlines, quizzes, review of videotapes for accuracy and clarity, and application for ANA-recognized continuing education units (if desired), among other activities.

   As per our discussion, specific content to be included in classroom presentation includes

   - physical and psychological assessment of the orthopedic patient,
   - emergency and intensive care of the patient with a spinal cord injury,
   - integrating care of orthopedic injuries into the total care plan for a critically ill or traumatized patient,

- motorcycle trauma, and
- intraoperative care of the orthopedic patient

16.5 hours

7. Final test. Test is prepared, administered, and corrected; results are collated; feedback is provided to group; and recommendations are generated.

8.0 hours

8. Communication with staff nurses and doctors. In addition to the introductory/explanatory time in activity 1, eight hours of verbal and written communication time is built into the project to provide the time necessary for investigating problems, answering questions, complying with requests for assistance with special needs.

48.0 hours

9. Committee work and team building. This time is needed to build an orthopedic team that will serve as the nucleus for development of solutions to future and ongoing nurse practice needs. The team will be prepared to deal with standards of nursing care with patients of increased complexity, nursing forms, teaching tools, policies, and procedures. In addition to the contribution made to departmental management, these activities contribute to staff's sense of achievement and recognition, thereby improving motivation and productivity. This approach to orthopedic content also makes it impossible for the departure of one staff member to take away all the institution's orthopedic expertise. Projects of other sorts (quality assurance, for example) can be assigned to the team as a working group, or the team can be used as a model to spread this approach to other in-house projects. The early sessions are aimed at encouraging group/team development, offering technical

	assistance, providing expert input, and supporting group and change process.
32.0 hours	10. Review of committee-developed output. Evaluation, recommendations, input, reinforcement, encouragement, and support are provided.
10.0 hours	11. Interim progress reports and strategy meetings with nursing administration. These communication efforts, amounting to ten hours spread throughout the project, will direct the course of the project.
10.5 hours	12. Termination of consulting relationship. This final phase involves reviewing progress, preparing a final report, and meeting to present the final report and recommendations. If desired, preparation of CEU certificates can be included here. This phase could logically include assistance with development and implementation of strategies to recoup return on investment.

1986–1987 Fee Schedule

Hourly Rate	Total Project Time
$75.00/hour	Any portion of an hour through 239 hours
$62.50/hour	240–479 hours: entire project billed at $62.50/hour
$50.00/hour	480 or more hours: entire project billed at $50.00/hour

Fees are to be paid in thirds: one third is due and payable on signing of the contract (invoice attached); on third is payable midway through the project (invoice will be sent); and one third is payable on completion of the project (invoice will be sent). Approximately four months will be needed for completion of the project: The project's hours may be extended beyond the four-month time period, if this is necessary to achieve maximum results for the client.

Consultant-incurred expenses directly attributable to this project are the responsibility of the client. Such expenses may include, but are not limited to, the purchase or rental of educational materials (books, movies) and computerized literature searches. If expenses are incurred, invoices and documentation will be submitted on a monthly basis.

For the duration of the project, the client is to provide the consultant with locked office space, office supplies, a beeper, a telephone, a listing of telephone numbers and the locations of nursing service managers, secretarial support, photocopy capabilities, an incoming mailbox (located with or near other nursing service mailers), audiovisual supplies and services (preparation of slides; shooting of videotapes; use of projectors, overheads, and other such equipment, as required), free parking, and access to cafeteria services.

In the event of inclement weather or illness necessitating the cancellation of a scheduled session or sessions, rescheduling will be done at a mutually acceptable time.

hours @ $ /hour =

____

Total duration of project in hours — Cost of project

I hereby accept the terms and conditions of this contract. Please sign and return one copy, and keep one copy for your records.

______________________________ ______________

Hospital (signature of authorized hospital representative) — Date

______________________________ ______________

Advanced Health Care Concepts
Nancy Doleysh, MSN, RN
President — Date

Appendix F SAMPLE SUBCONTRACT

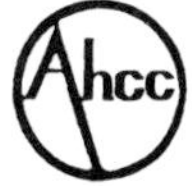

ADVANCED HEALTH CARE CONCEPTS

3799 TURNWOOD DRIVE, RICHFIELD, WISCONSIN 53076

PROGRAM ____________________

NAME ____________________

Present position:

Specialty area:

University:

Highest degree:

CONTRACT

You have indicated your willingness to participate in the above-named program, sponsored by Advanced Health Care Concepts, at

Date: ____________ Time: ____________

Location: ____________

Your compensation for the services agreed upon will be ______ to be paid within 30 days after the presentation.

In order for AHCC to present this course, advanced registration of ______ persons is necessary. Otherwise, the program will be cancelled, and this agreement shall be invalid.

Please sign and return the white copy by ____________

to ____________

Signature: ____________

Date: ____________

____

AV REQUEST

To ensure availability of the audiovisual equipment you require, please complete this part of the form.

__________ Overhead projector

__________ Blank transparencies/pens

__________ 35-mm slide projector

__________ Blank carousel

__________ Screen

__________ Other ____

In order to ensure duplication of materials necessary for distribution to the participants, please submit the materials

to ____

by ____

Appendix G RESOURCE LISTING

The following list is a compilation of the resources cited in the text.

PROFESSIONAL NURSING RESOURCES

American Nurses Association, Inc.
2420 Pershing Road
Kansas City, MO 64108
(816) 474-5720

American Nurses Association, Inc.
Washington Office
1101 14th St. NW, Suite 200
Washington, DC 20005
(202) 789-1800

National Center for Nursing Research
Building 38A, Room B2E17
Bethesda, MD 20894
(301) 496-0256

National League for Nursing
10 Columbus Circle
New York, NY 10019
(212) 582-1022

For information regarding the film *Breaking Down the Barriers to Nursing Practice*, contact the League at (800) 847-8480 or, in New York State, (800) 442-4516.

Nurse Consultants Association, Inc.
414 Plaza Dr.
Suite 209
Westmont, IL 60559
(312) 655-0087

SMALL BUSINESS INFORMATION AND FINANCE RESOURCES

Donor's Forum
208 LaSalle Street
Chicago, IL 60654

The Foundation Center
888 Seventh Avenue
New York, NY 10019

The Foundation Center
10001 Connecticut Avenue NW
Washington, DC 20036

The National Venture Capital Association
1655 North Fort Meyer Drive, Suite 700
Arlington, VA 22209

Small Business Administration
Financial Assistance Division
Office of Lender Relations
Non-Bank Lender Section
Washington, DC 20416

US Securities and Exchange Commission
450 Fifth Street NW
Washington, DC 20549

You may obtain the brochure *Q&A: Small Business and the SEC* from this organization.

INDEX

Assessment, self-
business and management skills, 50–51
critical events, 41–43
entrepreneurial orientation inventory, 36–41
interpersonal skills, 49–50
nursing expertise, 52–53
personal characteristics, 43–48

Bank loans. *See* Financing
Budget. *See* Financial documents

Change, organizational
culture and, 254–255
resistance to, 250–253
roles in, 248
stages in process of 249–250
Consultant
roles, 228–231
skills, 231–233
Consulting
contracts, 237–240
phases of, 223–228
proposals, 234–237
Contributions, of nurse entrepreneurs
to nurses and nursing, 261–264
to patients, 259–261

Developing a business idea
contacting role models, 62
focusing on one idea at a time, 62
goals, 66–68
launching a trial balloon, 98–99
making it unique, 62
personal skills related to, 56–62

Entrepreneur
career path of, 23–26
definitions of, 3–4
Entrepreneurial personality
characteristics of, 26–32
gender differences and, 32–35
self-assessment exercises for, 35–53
Entrepreneurial role. *See also* Nursing and health care trends; Socioeconomic trends
advantages and disadvantages of, 16–21
Equipment and supplies, for a business, 143–145

Financial documents
balance sheets, 197–202
break-even analysis, 204–207
budget, 194–197
budget deviation analysis, 197–198
cash flow schedule, 202–203
income statements, 197–202
personal financial statement, 189–194
Financial mistakes, common, 207–208
Financing
bank loans, 174–176
characteristics that appeal to investors, 217–218
foundations as source of, 178
growth, 217–219
national center for nursing research as a source of, 180
small business association funding, 176–178
start up, examples of, 174–176
state and local agency funding, 178
venture capital, 178–179
Form, choosing a business

corporation, 131–132
partnership, 129–130
sole proprietorship, 128
Growth, business
planning the pace of, 209–210, 217
potential areas for, 214–216
Image, creating a business, 133–134
Market-service analysis
client-centered business focus, selection of, 83–85
client-centered needs analysis 81–83
data collection for, 70–75
problem identification, 75–81
Market testing
inexpensive methods for, 95–97
a product, 94
a service, 88–94
steps in client decision to purchase, 85–87
Marketing
advantages and disadvantages of common strategies, 160–161
basic concepts of, 155–156
components of a marketing plan, 168–172
relationship of variables to nursing businesses, 156–160
Name, selecting a business, 135–138
Nursing and health care trends
consumer awareness, 14–15
empowerment of nursing, 12–13
high tech–high touch, 13–14
restructuring of provider organizations, 15–16
shifts in acuity, 14
Office space
home office, 138–140
identity plan, 142
incubators, 142
traditional office, 140–141
Organizational analysis. *See also* Change, organizational
components of, 241–242
status of nursing in, 246–248
subsystems in, 242–246
Organizing a business start up. *See also* Equipment and supplies; Image, creating an; Name, selecting a business; Office space; Philosophy, developing of a business
checklist, key decision, 124
documentation process, developing, 148–150
goals as a factor in, 127
work process, developing an organized, 146–147
Personality characteristics. *See* Entrepreneurial personality, characteristics of
Philosophy, development of a business
business orientation, related to, 125
client relationships, impact on, 125–126
code of ethics and, 123–125
organizational climate and, 126–127
Planning, new business
benefits of a written plan, 105–106
components of a business plan, 106–113
issues affecting a nursing business, 113–115
research and resources in, 113–119
Quality Assurance
in education and consulting, 213
in private practice, 212–213
process of, 210–212
Self-assessment. *See* Assessment, self
Socioeconomic trends
corporate focus on entrepreneurship, 7–8
educational and informational support, 8
information society, 11–12
pro-entrepreneurial economy, 5–7
women's issues, 8–11
Trends. *See* Nursing and health care trends; Socioeconomic trends
Venture capital. *See* Financing